Blabber Mouth!

77 Secrets

Only Your Mouth Can Tell You
To Live a Healthier, Happier, Sexier Life

Susan Smallegan Maples, DDS, MSBA
& Diana Kightlinger DeCouteau, MA

BlabberMouth! Press
Michigan • Montana
2015

D0104698

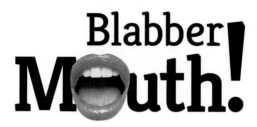

Library of Congress Cataloging-in-Publication Data is available.

ISBN 978-0-9963800-0-3

BlabberMouth! books are available at special discounts when purchased in bulk for premiums and sales promotions as well as for fund-raising or educational use. Special editions or book excerpts can also be created to specification. For details, contact BlabberMouth! Press at info@blabbermouthbooks.com.

BlabberMouth! Press

Printed in the United State of America

Second printing July 2015

10 9 8 7 6 5 4 3 2

This book is for informational purposes only. Consults your dentist or physician for all oral and systemic health issues. The author and the publisher expressly disclaim responsibility for any adverse effects arising from the use or application of the information contained in this book.

Cover design by Deon Staffelbach.
Interior design by Infinity Graphics.
Printing by Infinity Graphics.
Illustrations by Claire E. Nee.

DEDICATION

Susan dedicates **BlabberMouth!** to her mother,
Marilyn Sylvan Thompson, her father, James Smallegan
and her bonus-mom Dorothy Smallegan,
all of whom gave her the inspiration and courage
to follow her dreams

Diana dedicates **BlabberMouth!** to her father,
Gerald Eugene Kightlinger, who always wanted
to read a book his daughter had written

Blabber Mouth!

TABLE OF CONTENTS

Blabber Mouth!

PREFACE

Dr. Susan

DURING MY 30-YEAR ADVENTURE as a practicing dentist, I've become more and more concerned about the declining health of my patients and our population as a whole. I love my patients and attach my heartstrings to theirs, but I watch them, stand-ins for Americans everywhere, become fatter, more sedentary, more diseased, more medicated and more depressed—in spite of major advancements in science and medicine. Not to act is not to care.

Well, I care! So I have turned my concern into passion, my free time into learning, my frustration into creativity. This book is one of my attempts to "*be the change I want to see in the world.*" (Thank you, Mahatma Gandhi.)

As often happens when you pursue change, you find out how much you don't know—and just how wrong you've been. When I was a just a child, my Gramma Kitty taught me to question what I hold to be true. She often laughed so hard that her dentures would fly out onto her lap or she would pee her pants—but she was also wise in ways I barely understood. She asked my brother and me to memorize a poem she had taped on her refrigerator, a tenet that guided her life:

> *You're sure you're right,*
> *How fine and strong.*
> *But were you ever just as sure ...*
> *and wrong?*

As a dentist, I've always strived to communicate with confidence the truth about my patients' problems and present solutions with predictable outcomes. Without confidence, patients can feel lost and sometimes hopeless. The hitch is that telling the confident *truth* is often the same as telling an honest *lie—because we just don't know the truth yet.*

When I graduated from University of Michigan School of Dentistry in 1985, we thought that the mouth was its own private space. We thought that not much of what went on in there was linked to the rest of the body—and vice versa. Now I can't believe we *ever* thought that way. It doesn't even make common sense.

Signs of the most prevalent diseases we encounter today, the ones that result from unhealthy lifestyle choices and a sugared-up food supply, show up in abundance inside the mouth, making it impossible to ignore the many connections between oral disease and systemic disease.

Even the evidence revolutionizing our understanding of ages-old tooth and gum diseases is staggering …

We didn't know that tooth decay was a bacterial infection passed to babies, usually from their moms and dads …

We didn't know that gum disease not only resulted in tooth loss but also was a major risk factor for heart attack and stroke …

We didn't know that persistent human papillomavirus infection from oral sex would replace smoking as the single biggest risk factor for oral and pharyngeal cancer …

We didn't even recognize diabetes or smoking as big risk factors for gum disease—or suspect that gum disease made controlling diabetes far more difficult.

And the list of what we didn't know and what we got wrong goes on and on.

As a lover of dentistry and a learner with insatiable enthusiasm, I've been thrilled to put the pieces together that link mouth and body health. That's matched by a passion to save my patients' lives—and yours! But rescuing my patients, one at a time, inside the four walls of my office seems too small. So this book goes big, in the hopes of saving hundreds of thousands of people from the poor health that plagues countries around the globe.

I want to dedicate part of this book to my deceased father, Jim Smallegan, who was a fun-loving, wise and principled icon in my life. Here's his "mouth story":

We lost him 12 years ago, at the ripe young age of 73. Had he lived longer, he would have had such a positive influence on my son's life. He died when Hunter was only 9 years old, but for the eight years before that Hunter could barely understand a word his grandfather said. My dad had suffered six strokes in those eight years, each one robbing him of more day-to-day function.

He would tell us, in his garbled tones, "Having a stroke sucks!" At the time I thought his strokes were smoking-related, because he had no other *known* risk factors. But curiously he continued to have one stroke after another, long after he gave up his cigarettes. Each one stole a little more of the man I knew.

Cigarettes also stole his teeth. Gum disease goes hand in hand with smoking, and that infection was an ongoing struggle for my dad. After his first disabling stroke, he was unable to be transported to my dental office for routine care. He

Blabber M🫦uth!

was also unable to clean his teeth by himself. By the end, his mouth infection made his breath smell like rotting meat and he had difficulty chewing any foods that were not highly refined. He grew skinny and weak, partly from his inability to chew.

So in my dad's honor, I established a goal in my practice to help at *least* 30 patients a year quit smoking, so they could avoid related gum disease. Then one day, only four years ago, I was sitting in a Cleveland Clinic classroom, in a course taught by two of my medical mentors, Drs. Bradley Bale and Amy Doneen. A chill went up my spine when I heard, for the first time, compelling evidence that my dad's strokes were likely caused not by the smoking but by the one risk factor we had never before considered—the gum disease itself.

Even today most medical practitioners think of the mouth as the dentist's private domain. When they ask you to say *Ahhhhhh*, they're usually looking right past your mouth to the back of your throat. So when I speak to the residents at our local hospital and share insights about the mouth-body connection, they are aghast. I know part of my purpose on this planet is to bridge the big gap between dentistry and medicine, so we can work together to improve your health.

I hope that in reading this book you will learn more about your mouth—and its connection to your overall health—than you ever imagined. I hope you'll use this knowledge to further engage with your healthcare team, from your dentist and hygienist to your primary care physician and specialists. And I hope this book will spur you on to become an active advocate for your own health and the health of your loved ones.—S.S.M.

Blabber Mouth!

Introduction

WHAT COULD YOU LEARN if only your mouth could blab about itself?

You could learn how to live a happier, healthier, sexier life. New evidence is popping up every day that your mouth gives you illuminating signs of health and disease in the body, if you pay attention.

Act on what your mouth tells you and you not only make it far more likely that you'll be flashing a great smile into your 80s and 90s—but you'll learn how to boost your health and avoid chronic illness that can decrease the quality and quantity of your life.

Here are just a few examples of signs and symptoms related to the mouth and the possible health threats they could be warning you about:

Sign or symptom	Possible health threat
More bleeding when brushing or flossing	Type 2 diabetes
Eroding enamel	Acid reflux, throat cancer
Pregnancy gingivitis	Pre-term delivery or stillbirth
Gum disease	Erectile dysfunction
Periodontitis	Depression (and vice versa)
Human papillomavirus	Oral cancer
Narrow throat opening	Obstructive sleep apnea
Gum infection	Heart attack or stroke

But the focus in **BlabberMouth!** is health, not disease! In engaging, often irreverent, *short* chapters, we cover the full spectrum of oral and total health, including *aha* illustrations and a Quickstart to health in every chapter to give you a springboard to wellness. And of course, we include the 77 Secrets, many of which will be news that can transform health for you and your family. Here's just a smattering of what you'll learn:

- How to avoid giving your children the bacteria that causes cavities
- Which vaccination will prevent the virus that's the #1 cause of oral cancer among young people
- What you can do to overcome your fear of the dentist
- How altering your meds can help you skip another round of cavities at 50+
- What drinks post the most serious threat for obesity, type 2 diabetes and tooth decay
- How basic oral hygiene can stop you from getting pneumonia after surgery
- Why diagnosing hard-to-treat cancers and other diseases may be as simple as spitting
- Which debilitating disease projected to affect one in three Americans can now be screened for in the dental office

BlabberMouth! brings you the experience and insight of Dr. Susan Maples, a 30-year clinician, and one of the top 25 women and one of the top eight innovators in U.S. dentistry. She is also the co-investigator on a recent award-winning study on diabetes detection in the dental office. Dr. Susan doesn't lead an ordinary dental practice—she leads a total health practice that incorporates the knowledge we share with you in **BlabberMouth!**

Her co-author, Diana Kightlinger DeCouteau, is a journalist, essayist and scientist who's written for everyone from the *Washington Post* to *Discovery*. Her specialty? Explaining complex concepts in words with no more than three syllables.

Your healthier, happier, sexier life is waiting. Find out how to live it from **BlabberMouth!**

SECTION 1

Mouthing Off

AT THE MOMENT WE'RE BORN, we do only two things really well: cry and suckle. We quickly learn that we can get almost everything we need via the mouth. For a time, the mouth becomes the most important part of our body—and stays that way until we discover the rest of ourselves. But who can blame us for having an oral fixation at the start?

Of course, for most of us that changes as our horizons expand. (If that hasn't happened for you, you're reading the wrong book.) Later you may forget how important your mouth still is. And that's one reason we wrote this book.

As we say on the cover, your mouth knows Secrets that only it can tell—and we promise you a healthier, happier and sexier life if you listen to your mouth, identify issues and treat them with the help of your dentist and physician. So what are those Secrets?

They're sprinkled throughout the chapters of this book, but you need to start with some basics. If you're like us, however, you may not have the patience to read every chapter in order. So here's what we recommend ...

Skip Chapter 1, The Healthy Mouth, until you're reading a later chapter and realize we're talking about parts you're not familiar with. Then go back and at least look at the pictures. Eventually you'll want to use this chapter as a checklist for oral health.

Read Chapter 2, Bacteria, because it's integral to understanding the association between oral health and overall health that's captured everyone's attention, from *Scientific American* to *Time* magazine, from *Oprah* to *Dr. Oz*. Plus it's got a really good Secret.

Then read Chapter 3, Gingivitis, because 90 percent of us have it, and Chapter 4, Periodontitis, because it's going to be talked about over and over in the first third of the book.

Although you're going to learn a lot about what can go wrong in the mouth, the good news is that almost all chronic diseases, including the ones that impact the

1

gums and teeth, are preventable. And if you already have them, you can slow them down.

So we won't just tell you the risks that oral diseases can pose to your total health—we'll also explain how you can manage and sometimes reverse your problems.

Your mouth ultimately can tell you more about your total health than any other part of your body. Listen carefully to what your mouth says, treat it well and you'll reap the benefits from head to toe.

BlabberM uth!

Chapter 1

The Healthy Mouth: An Inside Look

AT FIRST GLANCE, THIS MAY SEEM UNFAIR: Dr. Susan's practice rewards a small, elite group of patients with special privileges. Of her 2,800 patients, only 60 are even eligible to belong to the "80/20 Club." And every year, the dental team invites those special 60 to attend a special luncheon in their honor and bring along a guest.

So how do you get in? You must be at least 80 years old with 20 or more teeth.

Given that we usually start out with 32 teeth, you wouldn't think it would be a big deal to end up with at least 20 of them in your senior years. But most people don't.

Not surprisingly, even though the members of the club are in their eighties and nineties, most enjoy great overall health too. Dr. Susan's team notices that these individuals also seem exceptionally optimistic and positive compared to other elderly patients.

Why does having more teeth correlate with better health? Think about the most critical function of our teeth: chewing. Chewing is the first significant step in the digestion process, and one we often take for granted. But if you can keep your teeth in good working order throughout your life and chew effectively without pain, you can digest your food better than your same-age neighbor who's missing teeth.

If you can't chew, you swallow your food whole, absorb fewer micronutrients necessary for health and set up a cascade of stomach and intestinal problems. Because of this, people with poor chewing efficiency prefer softer, more processed foods than those who have their teeth—which means their bodies get cheated out of nutrition.

So keeping your teeth makes you healthier. But the converse is also true—elderly people with good general health find it easier to keep their teeth until they're 100! That's because they've generally avoided chronic sugar consumption, smoking and other addictions, and constant stress—and that's helped them also avoid obesity, diabetes, high blood pressure, immune system failure and the like.

It's as though they took to heart the quote attributed to George Burns but originally said by jazz star Eubie Blake way back in 1921: "If I'd known I was going to live this long, I'd have taken better care of myself."

How does this pay off in the mouth? Less tooth decay and gum disease, and fewer worn and fractured teeth. And that's just the start. Keep reading to learn what a healthy mouth should look like—and what that can do for you.

> ## "Secret
>
> Research shows that if you keep your teeth and gums healthy for a lifetime, you'll add years to your life span. Your total health and quality of life will also be better along the way. "

Characteristics of the healthy mouth

So what does a healthy mouth look like? Here's the rundown on the key parts Dr. Susan's team looks at to make sure her patients' oral health is up to par

Anatomy of a healthy mouth

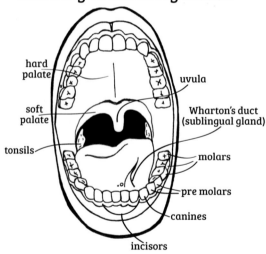

hard palate
soft palate
tonsils
uvula
Wharton's duct (sublingual gland)
molars
pre molars
canines
incisors

Lips: Your lips should be supple, with intact skin. The border of your lips, known as the vermillion border, should be clearly defined and not blurred by sun damage. You can easily close your lips when you aren't using your mouth, which keeps the interior wet.

Atmosphere: Speaking of wet, saliva counts. This has become a more critical marker of health, because saliva helps protect your teeth and gums. Saliva is a basic substance—and by that we mean anti-acidic—so it helps neutralize the mouth from the increasing acidity of our food supply. You'll learn more in Chapter 5, Tooth Decay, and Chapter 21, Cotton Mouth, about the critical role of saliva and what you can do to keep your mouth wet.

Cheeks: The inside of your cheeks should be wet and smooth, with no discolorations, hardened areas, abrasions or sores. In the middle of each cheek is a sticky-outy spout that opens the largest saliva gland, known as the parotid, into the mouth. If you push on the outside of your face just in front of your ear, you should be able to see that duct squirt out clear saliva.

Gums: The gum tissue that borders your teeth should be light in color—more like your face than your lips. Your gum border should also be tight and knife-edged against your teeth. This light, attached gum tissue should present a nice wide band. If you press on your gums, they should not turn white, bleed or produce pus. Healthy gums should *never* bleed—not even when you are brushing or flossing. Red, puffy gums that bleed easily put you at risk for many body ailments. Read more in Chapter 4, Periodontitis.

Between the gums and cheek: Next to the wide band of gum tissue attached to the teeth and bones is a zone of "unattached" gum tissue that transitions to your cheek. If you pull out your lower lip, about a half inch down you should be able to see a distinct line where the light-colored gum tissue becomes more red, thanks to an increasing number of blood vessels there. This tissue should look smooth, not ruffled, and have no discolored areas.

Tongue: Your tongue should be symmetric, meaning the right side should be a mirror image of the left, and smooth in contour, with small bumps all over the top of it. If you pull your tongue way out and check the very back of each side, you will see vertical ridges of tissue. These are normal but should be almost identical when you compare the two sides. On the very back of the top of the tongue (if you can see back there) is a row of round, mushroom-like bumps that are also normal. Again, make sure they all look alike from one side to the other.

Hard palate: Behind your upper teeth is another zone of attached gum tissue. Like all attached gum tissue, it should be light and uniform in color as well. The ridges toward the front, called *rugae*, help us pronounce words and propel food backward. The bulge just behind your front teeth is a large nerve bundle. You should not be able to bite into that with your lower teeth.

Soft palate: There is a line on the palate, behind which the tissue vibrates when you say *Ahhhh*. This is the soft, unattached palate and should be slightly deeper in color but still uniform. The hangy-down thing called a *uvula* is visible when you open wide and lift your palate.

Floor of the mouth: Under your tongue, in the floor of your mouth, you'll find a band of raised tissue that houses the biggest salivary gland—the *submandibular* (which literally means under the jaw). Submandibular or *Wharton's ducts* open on both sides of the midline and pour out over 60 percent of your total saliva. When they're healthy, with no ductal stones or infection, saliva flows clearly and freely. Saliva contains replenishing salts, so whenever these major pipelines open, the fluid can calcify accumulations of plaque, resulting in calculus or tartar buildup. Dr. Susan's hygienists call this pattern "salivary calculus."

Teeth: A healthy tooth has healthy layers. On the outside is the hardest, most protective layer, the *enamel*. Underneath the enamel is the *dentin*, a structure much softer and more elastic than enamel. The dentin is deeper in color and often feels "nervy" to touch or temperature when it's exposed. The inner chamber of the tooth is called the *pulp*. The pulp contains a hollow series of canals that carry the nerve and blood supply to the tooth. When this part of the tooth is sick, dying or dead, it can lead to severe pain and infection.

Anatomy of a healthy tooth

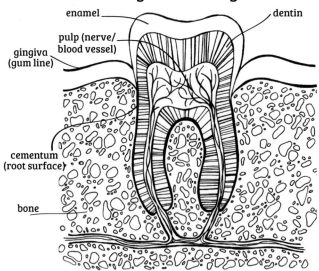

A tooth has one more key layer, the thin covering of the root known as the *cementum*. The cementum is easily abraded when the root surface is exposed. If you have gum recession, you are most likely looking at the inner layer, the dentin, rather than the cementum.

The healthiest teeth have no holes, no fillings and no discolorations. All the parts that are not covered by enamel are instead covered by gum tissue, with no root surfaces exposed. The enamel is not worn, chipped or fractured. All teeth are touching each other, side to side, and not so overlapped that they are hard to clean well.

Blabber M●**uth!**

Bite: The best bite relationship is when both upper and lower rows of teeth all touch together in perfect harmony. All teeth have a functional partner either above or below them. Front teeth are used for biting into food and back teeth for chewing. In your natural bite, as you guide your teeth forward, the front teeth ideally are the only ones touching. We call this guiding. When you slide your teeth side to side, ideally the canines (eye-teeth) are the ones guiding to their respective sides. In a stable bite you have no impacted or unerupted teeth and none of your teeth are missing. (You don't lose points for teeth missing to achieve a good orthodontic result or for wisdom teeth that had to be extracted.)

Throat: Using your cellphone flashlight app, try to see beyond your soft palate. This is the entry to the rest of your posterior pharynx and esophagus—the rest of your breathing and digestive tubes. You should see a nice wide, deep opening there. If the back of your throat is barely (or not at all) visible you are at a higher risk for obstructive sleep apnea or snoring, which you'll learn more about in Chapter 19, Obstructive Sleep Apnea, and Chapter 32, Snoring.

Tonsils: On each side of your soft palate are pillars of tissue (actually called the tonsilar pillars) that hold bulges of lymph tissue, which are your tonsils. An adult's tonsils should be small and not bulge into your breathing tube. They should also be smooth, rather than pockmarked, and not hold any globs of smelly food or calcified stones.

Temporomandibular joint (TMJ): This is the joint in front of your ear where the lower jaw and upper jaw fit into your head. When healthy, these joints both work smoothly without clicks, clunks, grinding noises or pain. Healthy joints have large and symmetric ranges of motion that allow us to take a big bite of an apple as well as to articulate speech and make wild facial expressions, something no other mammals on the planet can do. Learn more and see illustrations in Chapter 33, TMJ.

Muscles: Chewing muscles rule the roost. There is a saying in dentistry that "Muscles always win!" Chewing muscles operate opening and closing, from the hinge (TMJ) to where the teeth mesh. But muscles can get overworked and enlarged for many reasons. Large, in-charge muscles can result in broken teeth, shifting teeth, sore teeth, mobile teeth, TMJ pain and, yes, headaches. In fact, the majority of headaches people suffer are tension-related, from sore, overworked or spasming muscles. Muscles on the sides of the face should not be tender when you press on them or bulge when you clench your teeth. Compare your facial muscles with your biceps: Unless you've been pumping iron in the last 48 hours, you can squeeze your biceps hard without tension or tenderness. Healthy chewing muscles should feel the same.

Smell: Except for the temporary smell of foods like onions and garlic, your mouth should not have a distinctive odor. Any smell from your mouth is worth investigating. The smell may be coming from your throat, such as postnasal drip or acid reflux, the bacteria on your tongue, your blood gasses, such as ketosis from a drinking binge or uncontrolled diabetes, dental decay or, most often, from gum disease, which produces the putrid odor we call "perio" breath.

Quickstart to health

1. Get to know your own mouth.

Go through the list above and inspect your mouth carefully, identifying all the various structures.

2. Note any variations from the healthy mouth.

Better safe than sorry. If your mouth doesn't match our description, either we need better words or you need a second opinion. Take a "selfie" on your phone camera, so you have a communication tool you can use with your dentist.

3. Make an appointment to see your dentist.

If you see anything unusual in your mouth or haven't been examined in the past six months, it's time for a professional to take a look.

4. Perform an oral self-examination every month.

If you're looking at your mouth every month, you have a good chance of noticing anything unusual—even if it doesn't hurt.

5. See your dentist at least every six months.

Oral inspection doesn't take the place of a professional dental examination. Don't underestimate the care, skill and judgment of your dental team.

Chapter 2

BACTERIA: BILLIONS OF MOUTH DWELLERS

IT'S A REGULAR OCCURRENCE in Dr. Susan's office: a patient announcing in frustration that she must have inherited her mom's or dad's soft teeth.

Mom or Dad may be to blame, but it's probably not their DNA at fault. Go back to the day you were born …

Pouty lips, tiny flickering tongue, gums that would erupt in pearly teeth in months to come—your mouth was not only precious, but also surprisingly pure. In fact, at birth it was completely sterile.

But that doesn't last long. Even before you get your first tooth, hundreds of bacteria species nestle in cushy little crevices on your tongue, just waiting to colonize your teeth.

And where did the bacteria come from? Look to your loving and well-meaning caregivers, who licked off dropped pacifiers, shared silver baby spoons and planted the occasional sloppy wet kiss.

A study led by researchers at the University of Illinois compared salivary DNA in toothless infants and their moms or caregivers. The researchers identified a total of 397 species of bacteria, and only 28 were different between the adults and children. Among the bacteria most parents will probably transmit to their kids is *Streptococcus mutans (S. mutans for short)*, the bacteria that causes cavities.

> ❝ SECRET
>
> **Parents don't pass along bad teeth—they pass along bad bacteria not found in a baby's mouth at birth. To prevent tooth decay for a lifetime, don't share spoons, forks or toothbrushes with your baby or clean pacifiers with your own saliva until your child is at least age 3½.** ❞

9

Your own tropical island

Your mouth is home to billions and billions of bacteria, including those that cause tooth decay. They're joined by viruses, fungi and other bugs.

As you sit quietly reading these words, millions of microorganisms in your mouth are attached and growing on hard, slick surfaces like your teeth, fillings and dental appliances, as well as on cozy, cushy spots, like the tongue, cheeks and gums.

So far we have identified only about 700 different bacterial species in the human mouth, but estimates say the number is far higher, according to a study published in the *Journal of Bacteriology*. Not all of these are harmful bugs; in fact, most protect your mouth. But the bad bugs are truly bad—they are pernicious and destructive in the mouth and to the rest of your body.

Picture the mouth as a garden in a moist, warm climate you'd find on a tropical island. Many different bug species set up house within fractions of a millimeter of each other, but in separate communities determined by their needs, the other bug residents and the environment. Just like in a garden, the bacteria in your mouth compete with each other and, with regular brushing and flossing, many end up in your sink. Many more are swallowed.

In his book *Caries: A Treatable Infection*, Dr. Walter Loesche of the University of Michigan reported that the average person swallows about a liter (about the same size as a quart of milk) of saliva every day. Each milliliter contains about 100 million microbes. A little multiplication and we come up with the startling fact that we swallow about 100 billion microbes every day—which gives you an idea of how fast they're growing. No need to worry: Most of these bacteria meet their timely death in a boiling cauldron of stomach acid.

> **"** **SECRET**
>
> Our bodies are comprised of about 100 trillion human cells—and 10 times that many microbes, including bacteria, fungi and viruses, that live in, on and around us. The oral microbes play a pivotal role in our health. **"**

The good, bad and truly ugly

Before you get too weirded out by this discussion of bacteria, remember that a healthy mouth, just like a healthy gut, contains many species of bacteria living happily side by side—and in a mutually beneficial relationship with you, their host.

But some bacteria travel to other destinations, where they play havoc with parts of the body farflung from your kisser. Some are associated with life-threatening conditions, such as fetal infections, heart attack and stroke.

Others, like *S. mutans,* are scoundrels in your mouth. If your mama passed these bugs along, you need to take diligent care of your teeth and, perhaps more importantly, be careful not to feed the bugs frequently. They love to munch on sugary foods and drinks, and starchy carbs—and when they do, they become bullies. They spit acid on your teeth that makes holes in the enamel. The result is loss of tooth structure and possibly loss of teeth.

Dental caries is the #1 most prevalent childhood disease worldwide. And before you roll your eyes and say, "Well, every kid has cavities," realize that kids lose 51 million school hours a year due to dental decay, according to the National Children's Oral Health Foundation. And this is a worldwide problem. *The Sunday Times* in the United Kingdom reported on July 13, 2014, that tooth decay was the #1 reason why primary-school-aged children there were admitted to the hospital—to have multiple teeth extracted.

Remember we said that dental caries is the most prevalent childhood disease? If you love your children and want to save them from unnecessary pain and suffering—and the prospect of missing teeth when they reach the age of 20— know that caries is also 100 percent preventable if you can avoid bacterial infection and are consistent with dental care. We'll tell you more in Chapter 5, Tooth Decay.

Quickstart to health

1. Avoid swapping spit with your baby.

Although saliva has been shown to provide some protective benefits to children against development of asthma and eczema, dental research currently doesn't support the practice of introducing saliva intentionally. That's because of the risk of transferring organisms that contribute to cavities and periodontal disease.

2. Eat a healthy diet and limit between-meal snacks.

Remember what we said about not feeding the bugs? The bacteria that cause tooth decay love sugary drinks and foods, and starchy carbs—they chow down on these goodies and spit out acid. That's why you need to choose tooth-friendly between-meal drinks and snacks.

3. Brush your teeth at least twice a day and floss at least once a day.

You'll always have bacteria, viruses, yeast, fungi and other bugs in your mouth. But to keep their numbers lower and their colonies from getting more mature and severe, you can detach them by flossing and brushing, and then rinse them away.

4. Visit your dentist regularly.

With children, start even before they have teeth and definitely before the age of 1 year. And make sure you visit your dentist at least every six months and anytime you even think that you might have an oral health issue.

Chapter 3

GINGIVITIS: THE CANARY IN THE COAL MINE

YOU'VE HEARD THE SAYING, but did canaries really work in coal mines?

The fact is they did, well into the 20th century. Their job was to serve as an advance warning system for dangerous gases, like methane or carbon monoxide. Not only are canaries small and portable but, sadly for them, they're particularly sensitive to poisonous gases. The canaries would succumb to the toxins before the miners, giving the humans a chance to escape. Today the canary in the coal mine is idiomatic, an early indicator of trouble to come.

And that's much like gingivitis—an early indicator that serious gum disease could follow. But this gum infection is easy to ignore at the start, because it has signs but not symptoms.

What do we mean by that? Think of a *symptom* as something you feel (suffocation from poisonous gases) and a *sign* as something you see (a keeled-over canary). Usually it's the symptom of pain that tells you something is wrong with your body. But that's not true with gingivitis—it often doesn't hurt at all, unless you consider bad breath that undermines your personal relationships painful. So although up to 90 percent of people have gingivitis in one or more places in their mouth, with no symptoms to warn them, the infection often goes untreated.

What about the signs of gingivitis? The most common is inflamed gums, but we'll tell you about others below. First let's find out how the infection occurs.

> # " SECRET
>
> Gum infection, such as gingivitis, doesn't hurt like most other infections in the body. But if your gums are inflamed, you need to take action before you succumb to more serious gum disease that can compromise your entire immune system. "

How gingivitis happens

Surrounding each of your teeth is a cuff of gum tissue. This tissue sits right on top of a constantly forming plaque layer. If you don't do a good job of removing the plaque, the bacteria in it gang up and invade the gums. The gums respond with a full-body alarm.

To the rescue comes your 24/7 immune patrol, the white blood cells, to clean up the invasion. They travel through engorged capillaries that also carry red blood cells. That's what causes the reddish hue of inflamed gums.

What is inflammation? It's your immune system's response to insult. In the case of gingivitis, the insult usually comes from an overload of bacteria, especially if you are not doing a good job of removing it on a daily basis.

But bacteria may not be the only cause of your gingivitis. What if you get professional cleanings regularly, brush and floss on schedule and still have bleeding or red gums? It may be an allergic response to seemingly innocent substances like the flavoring in your toothpaste or foods such as gluten or red dye. Pollutants on tobacco leaves used in cigarettes are another potential source of toxicity. These allergens recruit your immune patrol just like bacteria does.

And if you have other diseases or medications that already tax your immunity, your gums may lose the ability to fight even small amounts of bacteria. Pregnancy gingivitis, a common condition for expecting mothers, provides a good example.

Warning signs of gingivitis

As we said, gingivitis does have signs, but you need to look for the out-of-the-ordinary. Certainly these signs should be uncommon for you:

• Reddish gums that match your lips instead of your cheeks;

• Bleeding from your gums when you floss or even when you brush;

• Teeth that look slightly longer where gums have receded and root surfaces are exposed;

• Recurring bad breath.

If you have a serious immune system disease—such as diabetes or HIV—or have chronic dry mouth from medications, smoking, radiation therapy, cancer, Sjögren's syndrome or another illness, you're much more susceptible to gingivitis. But here's the good news: At this early stage of gum disease, you can still get out of the coal mine alive if you act quickly.

From bad to worse

Many dentists and hygienists take an almost casual approach to gingivitis—after all, they see the signs we just listed every day. So they become concerned only when it progresses to periodontitis and bone loss, a more serious disease from both an oral and total health perspective. But no matter which infection you have, you need to take steps to treat it.

If you brush at least twice a day, if you floss at lease once, you can usually remove plaque. But it's persistent stuff—even if you remove it, plaque begins to grow back within a few hours.

Let's say you let it stay on your teeth longer than a day—even two or three—and the bacteria load gets heavy. You see gingivitis now, but also within 24 hours the heavy plaque can harden into tartar. (You'll see tartar used interchangeably with the word *calculus*, Greek for pebble.)

Tartar is almost impossible to remove without professional help. Both plaque and tartar form above *and underneath* the gumline. As the bacterial onslaught continues, it can cause enlargement of the gingiva, irritating and permanently damaging your gums. They swell, turn from healthy pink to sickly red, and begin unzipping from your teeth and bone, leaving root surfaces exposed and teeth unsupported. This we call periodontitis.

> # Secret
>
> If your gums bleed when you brush or floss, don't stop your routine. Bleeding is a natural response when you clean inflamed gums. Keep at it to reduce the bacteria load and avoid periodontitis, which is linked to a host of chronic diseases.

Restoring health

As we said, gingivitis is reversible. But do nothing about it and you will become acquainted with gingivitis' evil older sibling, periodontitis, and be at greater risk for many serious chronic diseases.

So even if the canary's feathers just look a bit ruffled, seek professional help. Be sure your dentist and hygienist are detailed in their examination of your gingiva. They will likely record a full "perio exam," including taking probing measurements and listing bleeding sites in response to probing. Work together with your dental team to thoroughly de-plaque your teeth and then thoroughly clean them on your own every single day. Within days your body will begin to heal your gingivitis and all those helpful white blood cells will go away.

If your gums don't shrink and return to a normal color quickly, you may need further care, such as a chlorhexidine antimicrobial rinse and/or further disease screening.

If your gingivitis persists despite good plaque control, eliminate potential allergens, one at a time, so you can gauge the difference. Start with changing to a toothpaste with a simple formula, like Crest original. If you are a smoker, stop it already: Many patients are allergic to one of the 4000+ chemicals included in the herbicide/pesticide cocktail mix on the leaves of tobacco.

Quickstart to health

1. Brush and floss.

No surprise here: You need to brush your teeth at least twice each day. Brushing with a spinning or sonic power brush will greatly help in plaque control. Floss thoroughly at least once each day, making sure to curve the floss into a C-shape and rub it up and down deep into the cuff of gum tissue until it meets resistance. Learn more in Chapter 35, Your Toothbrush, and Chapter 37, Your Floss.

2. Add a WaterPik to your hygiene routine.

A water jet really helps flush out free-floating bacteria and helps control gingivitis. But contrary to many of the advertisements, it will never take the place of flossing.

3. If your gums bleed, don't stop brushing and flossing.

No, you are not brushing and flossing too hard. Bleeding is a natural response when you clean inflamed gums. Keep at it, and the bleeding will subside as the bacteria load is cleaned up.

4. See your dentist.

Seek care right away if you suspect gingivitis. Also make sure you visit your dentist for a preventive appointment at least twice a year and get a complete assessment of your gum health and risk factors.

5. Address or eliminate contributing factors.

If you have uncontrolled diabetes, get medical help to address it. Diabetes is a risk factor for gum disease—and gum disease makes blood sugar harder to control.

If you have dry mouth, consider rinsing with saliva substitutes several times a day and/or suck on xylitol candies to increase saliva flow. But don't consume any sugar-laden candies or gums, or you'll soon have cavities too.

Learn more in Chapter 14, Diabetes, and Chapter 21, Cotton Mouth.

Chapter 4

Periodontitis: The Stealthy Enemy

WHEN YOU HEAR ABOUT LINKS BETWEEN ORAL HEALTH and systemic conditions from heart disease and stroke to diabetes to pregnancy complications, one word always comes up: *periodontitis.*

We'll state this straight up: We believe that avoiding and treating the gum disease known as periodontitis (or "perio" in the dentist's lingo) is the single most critical factor in maintaining your oral health—and a key to maintaining your total health too.

That's why this is one of the longest chapters in the book—because we want you to understand this stealthy enemy and what it can do to you. We want you to know who it impacts—and that's more than half of us—and how it does its dirty work. We want you to know how your dental team can help you fight back with diagnosis and treatment. And we want you and your friends and family to be able to screen yourselves for gum disease and let your dentist know if you suspect there's an issue.

In Chapter 3, we talked about gingivitis, the first stage of gum disease. But we've moved on now and the chronic inflammation has progressed. What can you expect from periodontitis?

How "perio" disease happens

In periodontitis, your firm, pink gum tissues now appear red, irritated and inflamed. The gums begin unzipping from the teeth, forming deep pockets underneath. You can't see the bacteria that fill these pockets, but they invade the gum tissue, causing it to bleed. Sometimes the pockets even produce pus.

Pus is an unsavory mixture of dead white blood cells, bacteria and tissue debris. Does this sound like toxic waste? In fact, it is. These toxins break down the connective tissue and bone that hold your teeth in your mouth. As the bone disappears, your teeth get a little loose and begin to drift, opening up spaces between them. That lets you save chunks of your dinner (and your breakfast and lunch) between your teeth. You might notice that your mouth tastes bad—and the people around you will definitely note an odor of rotten, dying flesh, a smell known as "perio" breath.

In the final stages of gum disease, your teeth might begin to abscess. That means more pus breaking down the last hold on your teeth. Your teeth may need to be removed or, if you're lucky, they'll fall out on their own and save you the dental bill.

After your teeth are gone, along with the bacteria, the body heals your gums. But without teeth to act as a framework, your jawbone keeps melting away. You may begin to look like a skeleton as your facial structure caves in.

Getting adequate nutrition becomes more and more difficult, because you can no longer chew the whole foods you once did. Now not only your oral health but also your total health is in jeopardy—and that's before we consider the link between perio and chronic diseases.

Perio on a rampage

Throughout the entire progression above, you probably experience little to no pain. No pain often means no awareness and no trigger for treatment. In the 1970s and 1980s, undiagnosed gum disease that led to a surprise loss of teeth was the #1 reason dentists were sued for malpractice. Today we have a fuller understanding of contributing factors—but we recognize that those factors are more complicated than we thought. So the disease rages on.

Periodontal disease progression

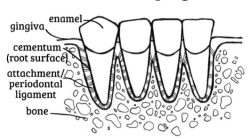

gingiva, enamel, cementum (root surface), attachment/ periodontal ligament, bone

Healthy gums and bone

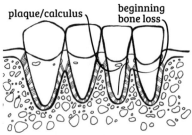

plaque/calculus, beginning bone loss

Beginning periodontal disease

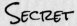

"SECRET

Periodontal disease is the #1 reason adults lose teeth. It's also linked to a host of chronic diseases—which means treating periodontitis may improve your overall health as much as changes in diet and exercise. "

How many Americans are stricken with periodontitis? The Centers for Disease Control and Prevention based their estimates on data collected as part of the 2009-2010 National Health and Nutrition Examination Survey. The news was not good.

Over 47 percent of the sample, representing 64.7 million adults, had periodontitis—and 38.5 percent of these had either moderate or severe disease. That number rose to 64 percent for adults aged 65 or older. It seems as Americans live longer and keep more of their teeth, perio also increases.

The study concluded that gum disease was higher in men than women (56.4 percent versus 38.4 percent), Mexican Americans, adults with less than a high school education, adults below 100 percent of the Federal Poverty Level and current smokers.

Worldwide severe periodontitis was the sixth most prevalent disease, affecting 743 million people, according to a study by the International and American Associations for Dental Research.

Because it doesn't hurt, many adults live with progressing disease for years, losing bone support and threatening total body health.

increased bone loss and increased root exposure

advanced bone loss that results in loose, drifting teeth and/or infection

Moderate periodontal disease   **Advanced periodontal disease**

The threat to total health

The questions you may be asking are *Why?* and *How?* Why does what goes on in your mouth impact the rest of your body? And how does that happen?

For decades scientists believed that gum disease was an isolated phenomenon. They knew it was the primary cause of adult tooth loss, but they thought that once teeth were gone the infection healed itself. Pull a festering sliver out of your finger and there's no long-term harm done. But that's not true for pulling a festering tooth out of your gums—it still poses a risk to your total health.

Periodontal infection—in short, invading bacteria—results in chronic system inflammation or CSI. By CSI, we mean a long-lasting, body-wide, hyper-response to try to heal the infection. It's no longer just about tooth loss, but about the threat of inflammation to every organ in your body. For more detail on how that works, take a look at Section 3 on The Chronic Connection.

Diagnosing periodontal disease

Before we talk in detail about diagnosing perio, be aware that clinical data just measure the damage gum disease has already done. So by the time you're diagnosed with the disease, your immune system is already fighting it—meaning you're already experiencing the inflammation that can damage your organs. It's much better to launch a counterattack early.

So how do you know if you have gum disease?

Your dentist should provide a thorough perio exam at least once each year that includes "pocket" measurements using a probe around the cuff of each tooth. The cuff of a tooth is where the gum tissue attaches to the root surface. The exam sounds like this: 2-3-2, 2-3-4, 4-3-5 and so on. Each number represents the distance in millimeters (mm) from the top of the gumline to the bottom of the cuff.

Probing pocket depths

Good numbers in this series are 3 mm or less. Bad are 4 mm or more, which indicates you have bone loss. But just as important is how the tissue responds to the probing. If your hygienist removes the probe and the tissue bleeds, this indicates active gum disease, inflammation and bone loss. If she removes the probe and the tissue doesn't bleed, the depth may represent an inactive pocket from previous bone loss.

An inactive pocket still poses a risk, because active gum disease takes place at the deepest part of the pocket. The deeper the pocket, the harder it is to

Periodontal probing

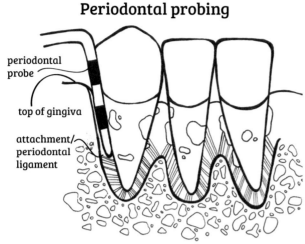

periodontal probe

top of gingiva

attachment/ periodontal ligament

clean and the more likely it harbors bacteria—which keeps the pocket at risk for re-activation. As a general rule, dentists can help you keep pockets 5 mm or less from getting any deeper if you take meticulous home care of your teeth, get professional cleanings every three months and quit smoking, if you have that nasty habit.

Even halting the growth of pockets 6 mm deep is possible but, beyond that, most pockets will continue to worsen. The only hope is to regain access for cleaning, often by surgery to reduce the pocket depth.

That's the clinical scoop. But dentists now have advanced ways to investigate periodontitis and treat it more predictably. These often rely on medical lab tests:

1. A genetic test looks for the protein interleukin to help determine if you are predisposed to gum disease. If your immune system is particularly aggressive toward inflammation, for example, you will want to be extra-vigilant about oral hygiene to prevent perio from gaining a gum-hold.

2. A saliva test for bacterial DNA can identify the presence of specific harmful bacteria in your gum infection, so the antibiotics recommended can be much more targeted. If you take the test before and after perio treatment, your dentist can gauge how effective the treatment has been. Learn more in Chapter 50, Salivary Diagnostics.

3. An A1C finger-stick blood test and fasting blood glucose test screens for diabetes and monitors blood sugar control. Why look for diabetes? If blood sugar is not under control, gum disease is harder to stop; and if gum disease is not treated, blood sugar is harder to control. Learn more in Chapter 14, Diabetes.

One more blood monitor you should be aware of is the high sensitivity C-reactive protein test (hsCRP or CRP for short). This test is often included with general blood tests at a lab. When your body experiences inflammation anywhere, CRP levels rise. Gum disease is one of the first places you should consider as the cause for inflammation, because you may not know you have it. Be sure to share information about higher CRP with your dentist immediately.

Your dentist will also consider compromising health factors that may put you at an increased risk of gum disease, including any diseases of the immune system, osteoporosis and certain medications.

From the chair

This is Dr. Susan and I'm going to dare to make a blanket statement:

If you are a regular smoker and over the age of 25, you will not avoid permanent bone loss in your mouth.

This disease progression often looks different than perio. In patients who do not have the other contributing factors for gum disease, such as poor oral hygiene, dental neglect, poor diet or diabetes, we often see bone loss without the typical red, puffy gums. The gum tissue can even be tight and light in color and associated with very little plaque or tartar formation.

Yet your bone loss still marches on over the years, and yes, you still lose teeth. We don't know yet how smoking destroys bone, but this much is clear: If you want to keep your pretty smile and chew whole foods all your life, quit smoking now.

Your risk of periodontal disease

To determine if you're at risk for periodontal disease, you can start with an assessment using Dr. Susan's self-screening tool. To take the test electronically or to share it with others, just go to http://SelfScreen.net or use the QR code below.

BlabberM😮uth!

Periodontal Disease Risk Assessment

Scoring: Yes=2 points, Occasionally=1 point, No=0 points

_____ Do your gums bleed when you brush or floss?

_____ Do your gums appear red? (Do they match your lips rather than your skin?)

_____ Do you suffer from bad breath?

_____ Do you have any loose teeth or teeth that have shifted?

_____ Do you smoke?

_____ Are there areas on your gums that get swollen or sore?

_____ Do you get food wedged between your teeth?

_____ Do you see exposed roots at the gumline?

_____ Are your teeth sensitive to cold temperatures?

_____ Have you ever been told you have "gingivitis," "bone loss" or "gum disease"?

_____ Has it been more than a year since your last professional dental cleaning?

_____ Have your parents or siblings lost teeth due to periodontal disease?

_____ **Total points**

Score total points:

0-3 Unlikely risk of periodontal disease: Learn more about prevention

4-7 Risk of localized periodontal disease/inflammation: Ask your dentist at your next visit

8-11 Moderate risk of generalized periodontal disease: Consult with your dentist asap

12+ High risk of generalized periodontal disease: Get immediate attention

Restoring health

With perio, we're way beyond the point where we can simply tell you to brush and floss and all will be well. Gum disease requires professional help.

After carefully weighing all the evidence, your dentist can recommend appropriate treatment options. Depending on the challenge your case presents, your dentist may refer you to a gum disease specialist called a periodontist. Your dentist can also help by working with your physician to manage any related medical conditions.

Your dentist or periodontist may recommend a variety of nonsurgical and/or surgical treatments:

1. Scaling and root planing: Remove the bacteria and calculus that initially caused the infection with hand and/or ultrasonic scalers.

2. Antimicrobial flush: Treat the gum pockets with a flush or localized antibiotics to reduce the infection.

3. Antimicrobial mouth rinse: Use an antimicrobial mouth rinse, such as chlorhexidine, as part of your daily cleaning routine.

4. Systemic antibiotics: Use targeted short-term antibiotics specific to the bacteria in the pockets.

5. Localized antibiotics: Place antibiotics in a chip or gel into pockets to clear out bacteria.

6. Reduce the pocket: Reduce the pocket depth with pocket reduction or flap surgery to provide better access for scaling and for daily home care.

7. Regenerate tissue: Reattach gum tissues after the infection is gone using grafting procedures by transferring a piece of your own tissue or inserting a substitute membrane.

8. Implant prosthetic teeth: Restore function and looks with new teeth that stay right in your mouth. Yes, even if you've lost teeth due to gum disease, you may still be a candidate for implants. In cases of severe bone loss, it may be necessary to add a graft of bone or tissue to prepare for implants.

Quickstart to health

1. Insist on an assessment of gum health at every dental appointment.

Make sure your dental practice checks your gums and pockets with a probe to identify any problem areas and conducts a thorough perio exam once a year.

2. Brush and floss and add a water jet.

You're never going to get away from brushing and flossing. But because pockets often make a little dip right between your teeth, the floss may not make it to the deepest part even if your skills are perfect. Add a water jet, also known as a Waterpik, to help flush out freestanding bacteria and reduce the inflammatory load. Learn more in Chapter 37, Your Floss.

3. Control diabetes.

If you are diabetic, work hard on your blood sugar control, which is crucial to heal tissues and halt gum disease. If you are not diabetic but have some risk factors, get tested. No matter what the outcome, work to improve your diet and exercise to prevent diabetes. Learn more in Chapter 14, Diabetes.

4. If you smoke, quit.

Even if you have no other gum disease risk factors, if you smoke you will lose bone support and end up with a jack-o'-lantern smile and difficulty eating.

5. Eat a healthy diet.

You've heard the adage "Garbage in, garbage out"? It's true. Your body's immunity to gum disease requires good nutrition. Micronutrients from whole foods serve as building blocks your cells use to fight disease and heal tissue.

6. Consult your dentist about options to maintain the health of your gums and bones.

Your dentist can advise you on diagnostic tests, lifestyle changes and clinical treatments that can help halt gum disease. This might include saliva testing, removing bacteria and calculus from your mouth, teaching you better skills for home care, reducing the depth of your gum pockets, grafting lost gum tissue and bone, and implanting prosthetic teeth to replace those you've lost.

Blabber Mouth!

SECTION 2

Tooth Decay, Disease and Death

In Section I, you learned how quickly a healthy mouth can succumb to gum disease without good oral health care—and how gum disease is linked to a number of serious chronic diseases that impact your entire body. But you may have noticed we skipped the teeth entirely. Trust us, we didn't forget. Unless you're under six months of age, gums without teeth don't support your oral health, function or beauty. And now tooth decay is also linked to serious chronic diseases.

That's why, at a minimum, you need to read Chapter 5, Tooth Decay in this section. Dental teams still fight a raging battle against tooth decay, even with all the advances in the last century. It's the #1 chronic disease that impacts children globally. And it's on the rise in a seemingly unlikely group—pre-schoolers. The high sugar and increasingly acidic American diet, coupled with poor brushing and flossing habits, put even baby teeth at risk.

And if you're 50 or over, make sure you take a look at Chapter 6, Root Decay. As you get into your fifties and beyond, your gums may begin to recede, especially if you haven't been flossing. This exposes your roots, which are seven times softer than your enamel. Decay can now proceed much faster, even to the point of damaging the pulp of your teeth.

The pulp, which is the living blood-and-nerve supply in the center chamber of your tooth, can't be repaired or replaced. When it's diseased or dying, your dentist will say the two words that strike fear in even the most stoic of patients: root canal. By replacing the dead pulp with a rubber compound, you get to keep the tooth for functional and aesthetic purposes. Learn more in Chapter 7, Pulp Damage.

But if all else fails—and sometimes it does—you lose the tooth. Yes, tooth loss occurs for many reasons, but among adults periodontal disease and tooth decay are the leading causes. Without all your teeth, you cannot chew properly, compromising the nutrition your body needs to be healthy and energetic. Chapter 8, Tooth Loss, tells you more about the harm to your entire body.

Consider this section a warning of the pitfalls that can occur without proper dental care—and a roadmap to avoid the most serious problems.

Chapter 5

Tooth Decay: The Price of the Sweet Life

You've heard the refrain of preventive dentistry all your life: If you take good care of your teeth and gums, and visit your dentist regularly, you can flash a beautiful smile that lasts a lifetime.

Sounds simple and yet, tooth decay is rampant. The Centers for Disease Control and Prevention call caries the most common chronic disease of youngsters aged 6 to 19 years. By the age of 5, approximately 40 percent of children have caries, and 8 percent of 2-year-olds have decay or fillings. Nine out of 10 of us over the age of 20 have cavities or missing or filled permanent teeth, according to the National Institutes of Health.

Even with all the tools at our disposal—an arsenal of toothbrushes, toothpastes, floss and mouth rinses, twice-yearly dental exams and regular cleanings, x-rays and perio probing—most of us can claim some tooth decay.

You can just imagine what your prehistoric ancestors' teeth looked like, without all the dental advancements and tools at their disposal.

Or can you? If he lived 1 million years ago to 10,000 years ago, your cave-grand-daddy (to the *nth* degree) actually had an extremely low incidence of cavities—less than 1 percent. Maybe he had a few spots on his teeth where the enamel was weakened, but no actual holes.

That continued through the Paleolithic and Neolithic, the Bronze and Iron Ages, despite the lack of so much as a toothbrush.

And then suddenly, from medieval to modern times, the incidence of dental decay exploded, reaching epic numbers in the 1800s.

The cause? A dietary change that amounted to a one-two punch. First came a switch from a hunter-gatherer diet high in meat and low in carbs to increased reliance on starchy grains like corn. That increased the incidence of lesions or holes where the enamel meets the root of a tooth.

And then came the introduction of sugar cane to the Western world, which resulted in a mouthful of cavities between teeth and on chewing surfaces.

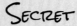

How tooth decay happens

What's needed for tooth decay to occur? Here are the ingredients:

Teeth. This almost goes without saying. Cavities form either in the outer layer known as the enamel or the inner layer called the dentin. Enamel is the hardest and most brittle substance in your body and also contains the highest percentage of mineral—96 percent calcium phosphate. The dentin underlying enamel is softer and serves as a moist, elastic support.

Fermentable carbohydrates. The carbs we're concerned about are sugars, like glucose, fructose or lactose—or they're starches that break down easily to sugars. By fermentable, we mean that bacteria can be used in the breakdown process.

Bacteria. If you read Chapter 2, Bacteria, you know there's no shortage of bacteria in your mouth. But tooth decay relies on a few species of bacteria in particular. One bug known as *Streptococcus mutans* gets things started; then its pal *Lactobacilli* helps keep the decay going. Remember from Chapter 2 that we are not born with these bugs; they're transmitted through saliva, mainly from our mom or dad. That explains why some of us are more cavity-prone than others. These cavity-causing bacteria take the carbs we eat and turn them into acids through the fermentation process. Without acid-producing bacteria, no decay develops. Likewise, without sugar and carbs, no decay develops.

Time. Tooth decay is a big acid-base chemistry experiment. It depends heavily on the amount of time your teeth spend in an acid bath. And we're not just talking about the acid the bacteria produce, but also the acidic beverages you may drink. (Coke, anyone?) Bathing your teeth in acid causes the minerals to leach out to buffer the acid. That sounds innocent enough, but it puts holes in your teeth wherever the acid pools the most.

The most critical factor in tooth decay is sugar consumption—but it's not how much sugar you eat, it's how often you eat it. So if you're going to drink juice or soda, think of it as an occasional treat and not an everyday staple. And when you drink it, suck it down, preferably with a meal where you are already consuming some kind of simple carbs. Do not sip this stuff. Sipping throughout the day means the bugs in your mouth are at an endless all-you-can-eat buffet, which lets them spit out acid all day long.

Warning signs

Tooth decay is a step-by-step process. The first sign that there's a problem is known as decalcification. This occurs before the cavities do and shows up as a white spot on your tooth. If the acidic environment doesn't change, the white spot grows.

We measure the acidity of the environment using pH, which ranges from 1 to 14. The lower numbers equate to higher acid levels, which might be the opposite of what you'd expect. So the saliva in your mouth is "neutral" at about 7. But add a Coke or Pepsi (pH 2.5), orange juice (pH 3.5) or Gatorade (pH 2.95) and the pH drops as the acidity climbs. Or more accurately, the pH plummets as the acid soars.

If the pH in your mouth falls to 5.5 or below, your teeth start to dissolve to neutralize the acid. The pH is a logarithmic scale, which means every whole number is a factor of 10 greater or less than the one above it. So Coke or Pepsi is 10 times more acidic than orange juice. It's not just a little more acidic—it's a lot more.

The white spot we mentioned above is a place where mineral content has dissolved out of the tooth. But tooth decay is reversible until you actually have a hole in your tooth. If you neutralize the acid in your mouth, remineralization can occur. Basically that means the minerals that leached out have been put back into the tooth.

Your risk of tooth decay

To determine if you're at risk for tooth decay, you can start with an assessment using Dr. Susan's self-screening tool. To take the test electronically or to share it with others, just go to http://SelfScreen.net or use the QR code below.

BlabberM●uth!

Tooth Decay Risk Assessment

Scoring: Yes=2 points, Occasionally=1 point, No=0 points

_____ Do your drink liquids other than water between meals more than two times daily?

_____ Do you feel like you have a dry mouth at any time of the day or night?

_____ Do you take medications daily?

_____ Have you had tooth decay and fillings in the past?

_____ Do you have visible white or brown spots on your teeth?

_____ Do you have any root surface exposure (gum recession)?

_____ Do you notice plaque build-up on your teeth between brushings?

_____ Do you skip flossing?

_____ Do you wear any oral appliances?

_____ Do you smoke?

_____ Do you have a history of radiation therapy or Sjögren's syndrome?

_____ Do you have heartburn (acid reflux or gastroesophageal reflux disease (GERD))?

_____ **Total points**

Score total points:

0-3 Unlikely risk of active tooth decay: Learn more about prevention

4-7 Low risk of active tooth decay: Ask your dentist at your next visit

8-11 Moderate risk of active tooth decay: Consult your dentist asap

12+ High risk of active tooth decay: Get immediate attention

Restoring health

So how can you encourage remineralization, so you don't get a cavity? Newer dental products that contain calcium phosphate, like MI Paste and CTX4 gel, help restore minerals. But you also have your very own secret weapon: saliva. Saliva is generally basic, the opposite of acidic, meaning it neutralizes the environment in the mouth and continually reinstates the minerals.

If your saliva flow drops for any reason, however, you're at greater risk for decay. One of the main reasons for decreased saliva is use of over-the-counter or prescription drugs. More than 400 of the most commonly prescribed medications—from antidepressants to antihistamines—reduce saliva flow as a side effect.

If your tooth continues to dissolve, the spot may eventually becomes "cavitated." The acid-producing bacteria move into the cave, where they're protected from your toothbrush bristles and floss. At that point, you'll need a dentist to fix the damage.

Your dentist will recommend filling any cavities, of course, but more importantly you need to work together to address the cause of tooth decay. Simply filling a hole without answering why it's there is like patching the roof over your bedroom to fix fire damage when there's still smoke pouring out of the living room. Instead you'd call the fire department, put out the fire completely, assess the damage and establish a restoration plan that includes future fire protection—all before starting the rebuilding process.

To predict how cavity-prone you are, dentists can now measure the acidity of the plaque on your teeth through a process called ATP (adenosine triphosphate) bioluminescence. They will also look at your personal risk factors, including dietary habits and disease history. Then you can decide on a treatment strategy personalized for you.

Quickstart to health

1. Brush and floss.

You knew we were going to say this. Be sure to brush twice a day following the directions in Chapter 35, Your Toothbrush. And floss at least once daily following the directions in Chapter 37, Your Floss.

2. Relieve dry mouth.

Dry mouth is a common side effect of many medications and a cause of decay when saliva cannot neutralize the acids in your mouth. Learn more about causes and treatment in Chapter 21, Cotton Mouth.

Blabber Mouth!

3. Change your eating habits.

Obviously we're going to recommend that you and your family keep your intake of sugar low. As you'll see in Chapter 43, Sugar, you'll need to be hyper-vigilant, because so many foods contain hidden sugar.

4. Limit acidic beverages.

The bacteria in your mouth already produce acid—you don't need to add to it. You're better off eating an orange than drinking orange juice and making soda a treat rather than an everyday habit. You can reduce the impact of acidic beverages by drinking through a straw and rinsing your mouth with water afterward. But don't brush right away—give your saliva at least half an hour to neutralize the acids and begin to re-mineralize your teeth first.

5. Consult your dentist.

Your dentist can characterize the plaque on your teeth, look at your dental history and consider your lifestyle risks for tooth decay—including diet, medications and home care. Together you can develop a treatment and protection plan that will work best for you.

6. Get professional fluoride treatments.

Fluoride lowers the susceptibility of your teeth to acid attack. If you are cavity-prone, take advantage of the professional fluoride varnish offered at your preventive cleaning appointments.

7. Chew gum or suck on mints/candies with xylitol.

Xylitol, derived from plants, is a natural sweetener that is a cavity fighter. It's been proven to constipate the bacteria in your mouth and keep them from spitting out acid onto your teeth.

8. Use a rinse or a paste with cavity-fighting ingredients.

Prescribed rinses or pastes contain ingredients like antibacterials to keep bacteria at bay, calcium phosphate to remineralize teeth, fluoride to protect enamel from the acid attack and xylitol to constipate the acid-spitting bacteria. In Dr. Susan's opinion, CariFree® offers the best cavity-fighting paste on the market, because it includes all these components. The professional strength can be purchased only through your dental office, however.

Chapter 6

ROOT DECAY: THE COST OF LIVING LONG

As you reach adulthood and pass through your thirties, into your forties and then your early fifties, your body begins changing in ways you might not entirely appreciate: lines etched on your face in the mirror, difficulty reading the suddenly miniscule print on restaurant menus, more tummy fat spilling over the top of your jeans, maybe even less interest in spending time awake in the bedroom. But on the plus side, your sweet tooth has diminished too and you haven't needed a filling in decades. So at least you're done with cavities—or so you think.

But as your fifties progress and you head into your sixties, you may be shocked to hear the "C" word again. This time the cavities aren't in the same place they were when you were younger—on the chewing surfaces of your molars or between your teeth. Now your dentist finds cavities on the root surfaces of your tooth, close to or under the gumline. This area is particularly susceptible to decay, because the cementum-dentin combination that makes up the root surface is seven times softer than the enamel that covers the rest of your tooth.

As people live longer and keep their teeth longer, they're more likely to suffer gum recession that exposes the root surface to the oral environment. As we noted in Chapter 4, Periodontitis, more than half of all adults experience gum disease—and that leaves the root unsupported and overexposed. Recession can also be a problem for people who grind their teeth, have bite-related interferences, have large and crowded teeth or simply brush their teeth so aggressively that they've literally scrubbed their gums away.

> ## Secret
>
> The risk of cavities actually increases as you pass 50, because receding gumlines and gum disease expose soft root surfaces that are more cavity-prone than enamel. All the good habits that helped you fight cavities when you were younger still apply.

How root decay happens

The most common culprit in root decay is gum disease from plaque below the gumline. When infected, the gums unzip, the bone melts away and the root surface is left naked to weather the new environment.

Enamel stops at the original gumline and the root surfaces beyond are covered with a thin layer of cementum. Cementum may sound like a hard substance, but its job is to attach your teeth to your jawbone, not to protect them from acid. In truth, cementum is soft, fragile and quickly brushed away. Cavity-causing bacteria colonize on the root surface just like they do on the enamel—but now they can attack much faster, because of the softer root surface.

That's bad, because without treatment the cavity can quickly spread to the inside of the tooth, where the pulp and nerve are. You may not notice the cavity until it causes a toothache or pain from infection. Or you may not notice a problem at all—our teeth become less sensitive as we age.

Because the root is so integral to the structure of your tooth, a cavity there can lead to serious problems. If your tooth is no longer structurally sound, it may break off at the root. Or if the root itself is damaged, you may eventually lose the tooth.

As patients become older or disabled, they may also have a harder time taking proper care of their teeth or chewing certain foods. If their diet shifts to softer, starchier foods, these will act just like sugar to cause cavities.

Warning signs of root decay

What are the signs that your roots might be decaying?

- Receding gums;
- Notches at the gumline;
- Discolored teeth, especially at the gumline;
- Holes or pits on the root surfaces or at the gumline;
- Toothache or pain;
- Abscess.

Root decay can be unseen, however, because it often hides just below the gumline or between teeth. Your dentist can determine if you have root decay during your regular dental exam. That's also why cavity-detecting "bite-wing" X-rays are so important as part of your dental treatment.

Your risk of root decay

To determine if you're at risk for root decay, you can start with an assessment using Dr. Susan's self-screening tool for tooth decay in Chapter 5, Tooth Decay. To take the test electronically or to share it with others, just go to http://SelfScreen.net or use the QR code provided.

Restoring health

If root decay is not too deep or extensive, your dentist may recommend a home regimen that includes fluoride. She may also suggest a calcium phosphate product to remineralize your teeth and antiseptics to reduce bacteria. It's possible with the right treatment to get closer to the hard, shiny surface you once had.

Your dentist may also get out a hand instrument or slow drill to remove softer tissue and then re-contour the root to make it solid and cleanable.

If a small cavity is already established, it's time for drill and fill. A larger cavity that poses the threat of fracture may require a full coverage crown. If the damage has moved on to the living part of the tooth, generally the choices are a root canal and then a crown, or extraction.

For a case where dry mouth is causing increased decay, your dentist may also recommend treatment to increase moisture in the mouth and replace saliva. Read more about treatment in Chapter 21, Cotton Mouth.

Quickstart to health

1. Brush and floss.

You knew we were going to say this. Be sure to brush twice a day following the directions in Chapter 35, Your Toothbrush. And floss at least once daily following the directions in Chapter 37, Your Floss.

2. Treat gum disease.

If you have gum disease, especially periodontitis, here's another reason to ask your dentist about treatment. Otherwise, root decay can compound the problems and also result in tooth loss.

3. Follow Steps 2-8 in Chapter 5, Tooth Decay.

Many of the same measures for prevention and treatment apply to both tooth decay and root decay, so you get a double bonus for taking these actions.

4. Consult your dentist.

If you notice any of the warning signs of root decay, schedule a visit with your dentist immediately. And if you don't notice signs of root decay? Visit regularly anyway to prevent problems.

Chapter 7

Pulp Damage and Death: Swan Song for a Tooth

At some point in our lives, many of us experience a tooth with a damaged or dying pulp. It's a problem as age-old as teeth. Happily, since the Middle Ages—and possibly even before—dentists offered any number of remedies. All you had to do is pick the option best for you:

- Remove the pulp and cover with gold leaf;

- Cauterize the exposed pulp with a heated instrument and cover with lead foil;

- Drain the pus from the pulp and call it a day;

- Pull the tooth.

We should mention one more detail: No matter which of these options you choose, the work will be performed without anesthesia.

Now doesn't that make you feel better about the modern root canal?

> ## Secret
>
> A cold-sensitive tooth does not signify a dying tooth like a heat-sensitive tooth does. Cold sensitivity can heal and reverse itself. Toothaches stimulated by heat or biting pressure or toothaches that appear without any stimulus at all are signs that your pulp is dying. You need a root canal to protect your body from infection and inflammation.

How root damage and death happens

To understand the progression of a damaged and dying tooth, let's start with the anatomy of *healthy* teeth. Imagine your teeth as hollow fence posts embedded in the ground. Beneath the posts are underground lifelines—a nerve and a blood vessel—that branch up into each post, giving it moisture and sensory perception. We call this the pulp.

A range of injuries and insults may cause inflammation in the nerve. Inflammation of the pulp is called—you guess it—*pulpitis*. Unlike an enamel defect, which does not heal, pulpitis can and usually does heal. But when it doesn't, the pulpitis advances and often causes a mama of a toothache as a sign of the pulp's passing.

So what kinds of insults can cause the nerve or blood supply to strangle and die? Trauma or fracture from a blow to the tooth, unbalanced biting forces in your jaws that disrupt bony support or cause a vertical crack, a high spot on a filling or crown, aggressive tooth grinding, tooth decay and even trauma from a dentist's drill.

Yes, you read that right: Every time Dr. Susan or any other dentist picks up a drill to help a tooth, she temporarily traumatizes the pulp. As you might guess, the deeper the cavity or more significant the fracture, the closer the drill comes to the pulp—and the higher the risk of permanent damage from the drill.

Warning signs that a tooth might be dying

Sometimes a tooth will be sensitive only to cold water or even air. This *reversible pulpitis* indicates the pulp is irritated but may heal in time. Your dentist can even promote the tooth's recovery by placing a soothing, sedative filling made from Eugonol or oil of cloves. Clove oil is the oldest remedy in the book for soothing the pulp, dating back to ancient Egypt. After giving the pulp six months or longer to heal, these temporary fillings can be replaced with the permanent variety.

That's the good news. But other signs of sensitivity or pain can indicate *irreversible pulpitis,* which requires a root canal or extraction. Irreversible pulpitis is marked by one or more of the following symptoms: sensitivity to tapping or chewing, heat sensitivity that stimulates a lasting toothache, or a toothache that has no apparent cause and goes away only temporarily with the help of pain medication.

Occasionally a tooth dies without any pain, resulting in either a calcified (solid) canal or in a painless abscess (pus sack) at the root tip. Your dentist can detect both of these conditions with an x-ray.

Most often an abscess hurts *until* the pressure of the multiplying bacteria causes it to push through the bone at the root tip and find a way to drain into your mouth. You might notice a little pimple on the gum tissue called a *fistula*. If facial swelling occurs, the infection is draining into the soft tissue instead of into your mouth. Even if the pimple or the swelling doesn't hurt, either one calls for immediate attention.

Leaving a growing infection in your mouth can cause big-time bone loss and threaten other body organs if the bacteria are travelers. We want to emphasize how dangerous it is to ignore signs and symptoms of pulp damage. Untreated pulp-related infections can spread and become life-threatening, especially if other conditions threaten your immune system.

Restoring health

The root canal is the answer to remove infected and inflamed pulp, sterilize the canal and fill it in. If you're squeamish, that may be as much as you want to know. But read on if you want the whole story.

Usually the procedure is easy for the patient. Either your regular dentist or a root canal specialist called an endodontist numbs the tooth, as he would for a filling. Then he will drill a small opening, about the size of the head of a straight pin, in the biting surface of the tooth and clean out the canal with thin files, removing all remnants of the pulp and infection.

Root Canal Progression

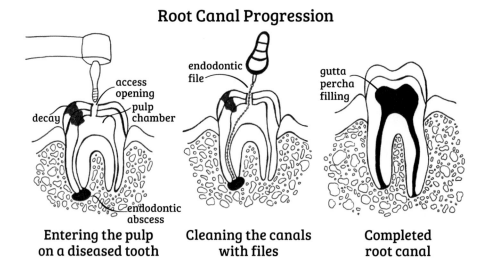

Entering the pulp on a diseased tooth

Cleaning the canals with files

Completed root canal

Canals can be maze-like, with multiple branches in multiple roots. The long-term success of a root canal, which depends entirely on *total* pulp removal, has increased through advanced technology—a microscope and live camera that guide the endodontist through the maze. Finally the canals are filled with a rubber-stopper-like material, *gutta percha*.

After "endo," the above-ground portion of the tooth must be adequately restored, often with a core buildup and a full coverage crown. Without it, the tooth becomes more fracture-prone, as it's now missing its moisture source and elasticity. In a tooth that already has been restored with a crown or doesn't require one, the small opening in the tooth must be filled to create a permanent seal.

Is there an alternative to a root canal? Yes—removal. In an abscessed tooth, it's often hard to numb the tooth sufficiently, because the anesthetic may not make it through the pus pocket at the root tip. But generally dentists are in the tooth-saving business: If a root canal is an option, your dentist will encourage one. A tooth with a root canal feels just like the rest of your teeth and, if permanently restored, can serve you for a lifetime.

Quickstart to health

1. Prevent tooth decay, and if you have it, treat it.

You know the drill (pun intended). Reduce your sugar consumption, brush at least twice a day, floss at least once. Although you can't prevent some of the causes of pulp damage, you can prevent tooth decay, the #1 precursor of a dying tooth.

2. Call your dentist if you have any tooth sensitivity.

Don't wait until your next regularly scheduled appointment! Often your dentist can help you avoid pulp damage by addressing sensitivity early. Relieving a bite interference, removing decay or placing a sedative filling are three examples. If the tooth requires a root canal, the sooner you have it the better, to avoid the spread of a more serious infection.

3. Wear a mouth guard when playing sports.

Any time you engage in contact sports or recreational activities that could result in a blow to the mouth, wear a mouth guard, preferably one custom-fitted to your teeth. One main cause of pulp damage or death is trauma. Mouth guards not only prevent pulp death but could also save your teeth.

Chapter 8

Tooth Loss: The End Game

From the chair

THE CAR SYLVIA DRIVES IS A RUST BUCKET *that looks like it should be hauled off to the junkyard soon. But then Sylvia is old too, and she's not a car person. Turns out, she's a tooth person. As a certifiable tooth geek myself, I applaud that.*

At 92, Sylvia still comes in for her regular dental exam with my team. Her hair is a bright silver but her dress is faded from years of wear. Still as the team often notices with 80/20 Club members—patients who are 80 years and older with 20 or more teeth—she enjoys significantly better health than most seniors 10 years younger.

But on that day, her visit with us would be longer than usual. I was replacing an implant crown on a lower back tooth.

Now you'd think by 92, most people wouldn't care much about a tooth, particularly one that doesn't even show when they smile. Most of us appreciate the aesthetic value of a beautiful smile, but far fewer understand the health value of treating gum disease or reinforcing back teeth.

Sylvia did—so much so that she was investing money she could have saved toward a newer car or other expenses.

"Why?" I asked. "Why is this tooth so important to you?"

She smiled. "I want to live all my days with a full complement of teeth," came the answer.

Sylvia is not alone. In fact, because you're reading this book, you've already demonstrated that you value health. Maybe you share more in common with Sylvia than your other friends would.

The very same week that I restored Sylvia's implant, I extracted an upper bicuspid—a visible tooth—on a 23-year-old man. He'll join the more common ranks of people who will be missing teeth well before they reach their senior years.

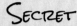

How tooth loss happens

Teeth are lost for a variety of reasons, from trauma to intentional extraction for orthodontics to removal of crowded-out wisdom teeth. But those aren't the main reasons for tooth loss. Instead most teeth succumb to periodontal disease or tooth or root decay—in other words, the progression of chronic oral diseases.

First, gum disease can destroy your gum tissues and eat away your jawbone, giving your teeth nothing to hang onto. Smokers and diabetics with uncontrolled blood sugar are particularly at risk.

Second, untreated tooth decay can create large holes in your teeth, resulting in a loss of structural integrity. Decay can also spread to the pulp, producing infection or abscess there.

And third, worn, cracked, fractured or broken teeth, especially when cracks spread vertically into the root, are also at risk for extraction.

A single missing tooth can also cause drifting, in which other teeth move either away from or into the gap where a tooth once resided. You may not notice drifting, because teeth move at the rate of glaciers. But bit by bit, drifting teeth can warp your bite, sometimes put harmful stress on your other teeth and even lead to periodontal disease. Spreading teeth also open up spaces between your other teeth, giving you a picket-fence look that might keep you from smiling your fullest.

Warning signs of tooth loss

As we said above, most adult tooth loss occurs due to gum disease or tooth decay, so you'll want to know what to look for. In general, you may be at risk if you experience any of the following signs:

• Loose teeth;

• Sensitive or painful teeth;

• Gum or jaw pain;

- Bleeding gums;

- Receding gums;

- Constant bad breath.

If you lose a tooth due to trauma, you may not have a warning sign besides the line drive flying into your face or your dog hitting your chin hard enough that your teeth slam together. Be sure your dentist knows when you've had tooth trauma even if all seems well. Although the tooth may look just fine, the tooth structure may be compromised. Traumatized teeth often die months or years after impact. They need to be monitored with pulp testing and x-rays to watch for death or a slow-growing abscess.

Restoring health

Like Sylvia, the average non-smoking adult today lives into their mid-eighties or beyond. No matter what your age, your overall health depends on your teeth—all of them—to digest the food that fuels your body and keeps you healthy and energetic. Chewing food is the first, and perhaps the most, important process of digestion. Front teeth cut food into pieces; back teeth smash the pieces into tiny morsels. Then your stomach can shred the nourishment into molecules for absorption. If you've lost back teeth, you'll probably notice that chewing with your front teeth puts them at risk for far greater damage. You may also be swallowing your sandwich in bite-sized pieces instead of well-mashed lumps.

So replacing broken or missing teeth may seem like a big expense now, but in the long run it will likely preserve your health, and help you save money and "save face."

Saving a tooth

If one of your teeth is knocked out, save it and take it to your dentist immediately. The faster you get help, the better the chance that your dentist can re-implant it. Pick up and hold the tooth only by the part you normally see, never by the root.

If the tooth is clean, try to put the tooth back in the socket where it came from. If it's not clean, rinse it thoroughly without scrubbing and reinsert it so that it is even with the other teeth. Biting down on a wet gauze pad or tissue will hold it in place.

If you can't find the socket to insert the tooth back in the gums—or doing that gives you the heebie-jeebies—put the tooth in a small container and keep it moist with saliva, milk or even water. If you feel certain you won't swallow the tooth, you can also transport it between the lower lip and gum or under the tongue. You may also want to consider a tooth-saving storage device as part of your first aid kit.

Don't worry if you are oozing blood. On the other hand, if blood is flowing in a stream from your mouth, apply direct pressure with a tissue or gauze to stem the flow. If you're in pain, a cold compress placed on the mouth and gums can ease pain. Also add an over-the-counter pain reliever, such as ibuprofen or acetaminophen, if you need more relief.

Replacing a tooth

We hope your dentist will be able to save your tooth. But if saving a tooth isn't possible or you need to have teeth extracted due to disease or decay, you have three alternatives for replacements.

The least expensive and quickest solution is a removable replacement: for one tooth, a flipper; for several teeth, a partial denture; and for all your teeth, a complete set of dentures that you take out to brush and sleep. Most patients feel more secure with teeth that never need to be removed, however.

A more permanent and traditional solution is a fixed bridge that replaces a tooth or two using support from the teeth next to the space. The support teeth are usually prepared for full-coverage crowns and the missing teeth are connected to and held up by these crowns. Your dentist then cements the bridge in place using the supporting crowns.

But bridges have disadvantages too. First your dentist must alter the support teeth, which causes unnecessary destruction of the enamel. Also it's not possible to floss between teeth in a fixed bridge, so extra time and skill are required to clean the sides of the support teeth using a floss "threader" or other gadget to protect them from gum disease and cavities.

The optimal solution is the dental implant, one of the great advances in dentistry over the past 40 years. These artificial root-like fixtures are inserted into your jawbone to replace one or more missing teeth or even to support a full denture. Ideally you have adequate bone to support the tooth and healthy gum tissues; if not, you may need surgery first to graft bone and/or tissue.

Which solution is right for you? Your overall and oral health, the quantity and quality of bone available, aesthetic requirements and financial situation will help you and your dentist determine the best option.

Quickstart to health

1. Treat gum disease and tooth decay.

Severe gum disease and tooth or root decay are the primary causes of tooth loss. Preventing and treating disease and decay are therefore the #1 way to ensure you'll leave this earth with all your teeth intact.

2. Wear mouth guards or helmets with face or mouth guards.

If you participate in organized sports or recreational activities, you're likely to take a blow to the face at some point. When that happens, you could easily end up with broken teeth and injuries to every other part, including lips, tongue, face or jaw. A custom-fitted mouth guard that fits over your upper teeth can help protect them.

3. Wear a bite splint or bite guard if you grind your teeth.

Talk with your dentist about a professionally made bite splint or night guard. Drug store mouth guards are soft like a dog toy—so you'll have a tendency to chew it. The excessive chewing forces could harm your temporomandibular joints (TMJs). Learn more in Chapter 34, Bruxism.

4. Don't use your teeth as tools.

Yes, they can pop a bottle top or cut a thread or even hold hangers, until they can't. Using your teeth as tools increases the chance of fracturing or breaking a tooth. So use them only to chew and then selectively—no frozen candy bars or ice, please.

5. Quit smoking.

If you don't stop smoking, you'll lose bone first and then teeth. If you've tried to quit smoking and can't, get help. Learn more in Chapter 42, Cigarettes and Chew.

6. Brush and floss.

Tooth loss is most often preventable with proper oral hygiene. And that means getting rid of food particles and nasty bacteria that cause gum disease and tooth decay. So brush at least twice a day and floss at least once.

7. Visit your dentist regularly.

The history of dentistry may have started with tooth extraction, but today dentists lean much more toward prevention and restoration. See your dentist regularly to address issues that might otherwise result in tooth loss.

SECTION 3

THE CHRONIC CONNECTION

IN 1989, A FINNISH DOCTOR named Kimmo Mattila and his colleagues reported on research they'd done on patients with acute myocardial infarction, what we'd call a heart attack. They noticed that heart attack victims they saw in the emergency room appeared to have particularly poor oral health. So the doctors conducted a study to compare the dental health of individuals who had—and had not—suffered a heart attack.

We'll tell you more about this study in Chapter 11, Heart Disease. But here's the upshot: Patients with a heart attack history had significantly worse oral health, even after adjusting for other factors that contribute to heart attacks.

The study sparked renewed interest among dentists and physicians on the relationship between oral health and total health. A new era had begun, one in which the dental and medical community united to research the links between the mouth and the body.

But why? Why would the health of your mouth make any difference to your heart? Or your brain? Why would gum disease, in particular, be a risk factor in diseases from stroke to diabetes to osteoporosis?

To date, two main mechanisms have been proposed, which we'll address in Chapter 9, Inflammation, and Chapter 10, Traveling Bacteria. The first mechanism says that infection triggers the immune system to fight back by releasing toxic chemicals into the bloodstream—and these chemicals cause inflammation that damages blood vessels and organs. The second suggests that bacteria from oral infections enter the bloodstream, travel to other parts of the body and set up a new home and the conditions for harm.

The two mechanisms overlap and work together. And although the relative contribution of each to systemic disease is not yet known, the story is slowly unfolding in one research study after another.

Chapter 9

INFLAMMATION: THE FIRE

Quit brushing and flossing for three weeks!

Those were the orders that 11 volunteers received from renowned dental professor Dr. Harold Löe and his colleagues. No, this wasn't some twisted dental experiment—rather the researchers wanted to see just how fast bacterial plaque would accumulate and produce gingivitis.

Turns out the answer is really fast. After only two days, the good bacteria in the subjects' mouths were joined by bad species.

In this case, the bad species were gram-negative bacteria—the ones you might have heard of because some are resistant to available antibiotics. That enables the gram-negative bacteria to cause dangerous infections, including those in the bloodstream, wounds and surgical sites. These bacteria may also cause meningitis and pneumonia.

As the experiment progressed, even more bacteria joined in, creating a community that didn't look much like the one there initially. At the same time the complex community developed, the dentists were able to clinically diagnose the onset of gingivitis, marked by red, puffy gums that bleed more easily.

In fact, 100 percent of the subjects developed gingivitis within 10 to 21 days. Mild inflammation began even earlier, probably with the development of plaque in the first few days. But when the researchers removed the plaque, the inflammation disappeared the next day.

What if the researchers hadn't reversed the experiment? Then the acute inflammation would have become chronic, which is even more dangerous.

> **" SECRET**
>
> The amount of plaque in your mouth matters, but so does its age. Plaque that's in your mouth for 24 hours or more harbors more dangerous bacteria, so clean your teeth every day. **"**

Blabber Mouth!

How inflammation helps and harms us

Until our last breath on earth, our bodies are constantly at work, striving against all odds to heal from the barrage of threats it receives—from injury, infection, allergens, physical and chemical agents, tissue death, genetic defects and a host of other insults. Putting ourselves in an optimal state of health means we need to slow down the harmful insults and reduce inflammation throughout the system.

Dire as inflammation sounds—literally, "to kindle" or "to light on fire"—our bodies could not survive without it. Inflammation is our body's natural 24/7 protective mechanism, prompting helper cells to swoop in to clean up the initial cause of insults and to help heal them.

Let's take a quick look at acute inflammation, which is short in time, and focused on quick healing. An insult or injury—anything from a splinter to a cold virus to a burn—damages tissues. For example, let's assume you cut your finger with a knife while slicing tomatoes.

Bacteria immediately invade the cut—and that prompts nearby cells to send an alarm recruiting helper immune cells to the site. The first responders are local white blood cells known as macrophages—literally the big, sloppy eaters. They get to work gobbling up bacteria, while waiting on other white blood cells to arrive via the bloodstream.

To make a pathway for the traveling cells, the macrophages release chemicals that widen the local blood vessels. This extra blood is where the redness, swelling, heat and pain that inflame the area come from. You can even experience loss of function if the inflammatory response is dramatic enough.

Dendritic cells within the tissues provide information on the invading organism to identify the threat and call in the appropriate agents. You don't bring a knife to a gunfight; likewise your body doesn't fight a splinter in the same way it fights a cold.

Now your infected cut calls for the help of white blood cells known as neutrophils. The neutrophils are filled with tiny sacs that contain enzymes to digest microorganisms.

To keep all the comings and goings orderly, the entire inflammatory response is coordinated by cytokines. Cytokines are proteins in your body that act as chemical mediators, sending signals between immune cells. The goal ultimately is to clear up the insult—in this case, the invading bacteria—and repair the tissue.

Once the enemy organism is defeated, the fighting cells leave via the bloodstream and the dead cells are taken away. The fibroblasts—think of them as construction workers—go to work repairing the tissue. The body heals and the inflammatory process turns off.

Except when it doesn't.

What if the inflammatory process continues or goes into overdrive? Say you're walking around with untreated gum disease. Or you have an unknown food sensitivity to gluten or dairy. Or you're exposed daily to a personal toxin, such as a food additive, pesticide or prescription medication. Or your immune system is out of whack and reacts to a harmless agent in the same way it would to a real problem.

Then you're looking at chronic systemic inflammation (CSI).

By chronic, we mean long-lasting.

By systemic, we mean throughout your entire body.

And by inflammation, we mean a hyper-version of the response we described above.

Chronic systemic inflammation

In CSI, the body's immune response doesn't work as it should. Instead of quickly striking and resolving an insult, your immune system continues to release white blood cells and biochemical byproducts that damage your tissues, especially the linings of your blood vessels.

Drs. Bradley Bale and Amy Doneen, authors of *Beat the Heart Attack Gene,* call this a "fire" in the blood vessels. This weakness lets traveling oral bacteria from gum disease to penetrate the blood vessel wall. There the bacteria can build a nest, reproduce and eventually erupt—triggering a clot that could cause a heart attack or stroke.

The chemical mediators that are part of inflammation may also reach the liver, activating the production of proteins there. That's why one way to measure CSI is with a blood test called HsCRP (High Sensitivity C-Reactive Protein). This test will tell you if you're experiencing inflammation in the body, although it won't tell you where. But given the relationship between inflammation and cardiovascular disease, physicians use the HsCRP test to determine the risk of heart attack and stroke.

In addition to cardiovascular disease, uncontrolled CSI can lead to a litany of ailments from diabetes to pregnancy complications to periodontitis. That's why reducing levels of inflammatory markers may help reduce the risk of systemic diseases.

Your risk of chronic system inflammation

To determine if you're at risk for chronic system inflammation, you can start with an assessment using Dr. Susan's self-screening tool. To take the test electronically or to share it with others, just go to http://SelfScreen.net or use the QR code below.

Chronic System Inflammation Risk Assessment

Scoring: Yes=2 points, Occasionally=1 point, No=0 points

_____   Do you have a large waistline (above 35 inches for women and above 40 inches for men)?

_____   Do you have difficulty losing weight despite considerable effort?

_____   Do you suffer from inexplicably achy joints or sore muscles?

_____   Do you suffer from food sensitivities or gastrointestinal disturbances, such as discomfort, bloating, constipation or diarrhea?

_____   Do you have low energy and/or sleep problems?

_____   Do you have dry, patchy, red or irritated skin, itchy ears or itchy eyes?

_____   Do you have red, puffy or bleeding gums when you brush or floss, or do you suffer from constant bad breath?

_____   Do you smoke or take any medications (prescription or over-the-counter)?

_____   Do you have significant and persistent stress in your life?

_____   Do you have persistent unexplained nasal congestion?

_____   Do you have diabetes, hypertension or high cholesterol/lipid profile?

_____   Do you suffer from any chronic diseases?

_____   Do you exercise fewer than three times a week?

_____   **Total points**

Score total points:

0-5 Unlikely risk of CSI: Learn more about prevention

5-10 Moderate risk of CSI: Consult with your physician

10+ High risk of CSI: Get immediate attention

Quickstart to health

1. Address your gum health.

Make sure you visit your dentist regularly, get your gums assessed and treat any problems.

2. Brush and floss.

As Dr. Löe's research showed, reducing the bacterial load in your mouth and removing plaque can help curtail inflammation.

3. Lose weight if you're overweight or obese.

Studies by researchers at the Pennington Biomedical Research Center showed that men with higher body mass indexes have raised levels of inflammatory markers. Even losing a small amount of your body weight can make a major difference in your risk for CSI.

4. Try a short-term anti-inflammatory diet.

Avoid foods that might trigger CSI, such as dairy, gluten, sugar, caffeine and chemicals in processed foods, for 21 days. You might notice a big difference in how you feel. Then add back favorite foods, one at a time, to see if these trigger your signs of CSI from the self-screen.

5. Get fit.

Studies show that individuals who don't exercise have higher levels of inflammatory markers. Fight inflammation by exercising regularly.

6. Lower your stress levels and get adequate sleep.

Eat a healthy diet, reduce caffeine and sugar, limit alcohol, avoid tobacco and recreational drugs, and sleep seven to nine hours each night.

Chapter 10

TRAVELING BACTERIA: THE MOVEABLE INFECTION

VISIT YOUR DENTIST TODAY with a damaged, decaying or diseased tooth and one thing is almost certain: Your dentist will try to help you keep that tooth. That's because dentists today practice preventive and restorative dentistry.

But 100 years ago, if you'd visited the dentist, chances are you were in pain. And to stop that pain, your dentist would have given you the very good news that he was a 100 percenter. By that we mean that he would extract 100 percent of your teeth that were hurting or diseased.

The oral sepsis theory

Although pulling teeth instead of restoring them to health seems like a radical approach to us today, a century ago it made sense to practitioners. In 1891, a University of Pennsylvania Dental School graduate named Dr. Willoughby D. Miller published a report called *The Human Mouth as a Focus of Infection*.

Miller became convinced that bacteria in the mouth could explain most of humankind's illnesses. Given all the bacteria and other bugs found in the mouth, you might understand why Miller took this position. Basically a focus of infection is a confined area that contains disease-causing microorganisms. This focus can occur anywhere in the body, and usually causes no systemic trouble.

Miller proposed a role for microorganisms or their toxins in the development of diseases in sites nowhere near the mouth—everything from brain abscesses and lung diseases to stomach problems.

If Miller was right, what would fix the many diseases of the body? Extracting all diseased teeth, including those with cavities or nerve damage or surrounding gum disease. That would eliminate any possible focus of infection. Never mind that in an era when tooth brushing was just coming into vogue, almost everyone suffered from bad teeth and gums.

Eventually the lack of research on these links and therefore the lack of scientific evidence to support them led to the demise of the concept of focal infection. In fact, when Dr. Susan attended the highly ranked University of Michigan Dental School in the mid-1980s, she was taught that diseases in and around teeth were mostly isolated, except in instances where a local infection spread to nearby tissues.

But the connection between oral and overall health has made a strong comeback and the evidence continues to grow every day. Research that supports the links between oral health and total body health is mounting. And the leaders of every major dental school and professional organization know that learning more and practicing the mouth-body connection is dentistry's future.

Traveling bacteria: setting up infection

Scientists estimate that the number of bacteria we host on us and in us is 10 times more than the number of living cells in the body. Think of the character Pigpen in the old Charlie Brown comics. Like Pigpen, we literally walk around in a cloud of bugs. Most of them are not harmful and the ones that are don't do their dirty work unless the resistance of the host—that's us—is low.

We call it infection whenever a bacteria, virus or fungus invades your body. Intact skin serves as one of the body's best protections against microbes. In terms of our mouths, healthy, tight gums serve as that protection. But when our gums are bugged-up from poor oral hygiene, smoking, diabetes or another metabolic issue, the tissue becomes inflamed and fragile.

" SECRET

Stretch out the circumferences of all the gum tissue that surrounds your teeth and the line would extend from the tip of your index finger to the top of your shoulder. Preventing gum disease along that 24-inch length reduces the infection your body must fight and the risk of other chronic diseases. **"**

You'd never ignore a 2'-long cut on your arm—especially if it was teeming with bacteria—but millions of people pay no attention to the same phenomenon in their mouth. Puffy, red gums that bleed create a door through which dangerous bugs can enter the bloodstream.

Researchers once thought that transfer of bacteria into the bloodstream occurred most frequently during dental procedures. That's why dentists pre-medicate people with antibiotics before routine cleanings if they have replacement heart valves or joints. But recent evidence suggests that bacteria in patients with gum disease are even more likely to enter the blood during everyday events, such as chewing, toothbrushing and flossing.

Bacteria in a different "plaque"

Dr. Wenche Bornacki, a prominent oral health researcher, recently published a manuscript called "The Traveling Oral Microbiome." In it, Dr. Bornacki describes the evidence we have for mouth bacteria and bugs traveling directly and indirectly to a host of body sites, including the neck, brain, lungs, liver, pancreas, joints, vertebrae, vagina and gastrointestinal tract. They get there using many different means: aspiration—being sucked into the lungs, transfer into the bloodstream, direct contact between humans, shared items like pacifiers and spoons, and sneezes.

In 2011, a group of researchers conducted a study to see if bacteria from the mouth and/or the gut could end up in plaque—the kind that resides in the walls of blood vessels. They found species of two bacteria—*Veillonella* and *Streptococcus*—in the majority of the artery wall plaque samples. Even more intriguing, the heavier the combined load of these two species in the plaque, the heavier the load in the mouth and gut. Several other bacteria were also common between plaque and oral and gut samples.

As Dr. Bornacki notes, "These bacteria may contribute to further inflammation and eventual destabilization and rupture of the plaque, ultimately causing a heart attack or stroke."

But infections caused by traveling bacteria extend beyond cardiovascular disease. Y. W. Han and colleagues reported on a stillbirth caused by the oral bacteria *Fusobacterium nucleatum*. This sad outcome provided the first evidence that bacteria from a human mother's gum disease could move to the placenta and fetus, causing acute inflammation that resulted in the baby's death. This species was not found in the mother's vaginal or rectal bacteria. Read more about the impact of gum disease on pregnancy in Chapter 17, Pregnancy Complications.

As oral microbes move throughout the body and stimulate responses, it's not surprising that they're associated with various diseases, including cancers outside the oral cavity, respiratory disease and joint infections. You'll learn more about all of these in Sections 4 and 5.

Quickstart to health

1. Brush and floss.

No surprise here: Good oral hygiene will help cut the bacterial load, reduce inflammation and diminish the chance that bacteria will enter your bloodstream.

2. See your dentist.

Make sure that at least twice each year you get a professional cleaning and assessment of your gum health and risk factors.

3. Get professional treatment for active gingivitis and periodontitis.

Establishing a plan to get rid of any infection in your mouth will help reduce the opportunities for dangerous bugs to enter your bloodstream and migrate.

4. Boost your immune system to help fend off traveling bugs and health from infection.

Don't underestimate the other lifestyle improvements you can make to keep your host (you!) strong, including better nutrition, regular exercise, weight control, more rest and less stress.

BlabberMouth!

SECTION 4

THE ORAL ACCOMPLICE TO THE TOP 5 KILLERS

HEART DISEASE. CANCER. STROKE. DIABETES. LUNG DISEASE.

These are the Top 5 Killers in America. They're the guilty parties in two of every three deaths. And the top two killers—heart disease and cancer—are particularly prolific: They kill almost half of the Americans who die each year.

Yet dying may not be the worst of it. Here's what the afflicted may endure in the years before they finally die: heart palpitations, shortness of breath, fatigue, coughing, chest pain, fluid accumulation, excruciating pain, weakness and paralysis, kidney failure, blindness and amputation.

This is the dirty work the Top 5 Killers do. But you need to know something else about them: For the most part, the Top 5 Killers are all chronic *preventable* diseases. In fact, of the 10 causes of death in the United States in 2011, seven are chronic preventable diseases.

That means even if you have a family history of these diseases, you can take action that will prevent you from ever experiencing them and their debilitating impacts.

The Top 5 Killers are mostly lifestyle diseases, which means you can't hide behind bad genes. Changing your habits can keep you healthy and alive. Revamped habits include fueling your body with whole food instead of junk, moving your body every day instead of sitting in front of a screen for most of your waking hours, and staying within healthy limits for sugar, alcohol and caffeine. And if you smoke or chew tobacco, think of quitting or switching to a safer habit, like skydiving without a parachute.

But we need to focus on one other key aspect of prevention, because there's strong evidence that poor oral health is an accomplice in *all* these diseases.

The evidence started building back in the 1980s, when a Finnish doctor and his colleagues realized that patients admitted to the emergency room for heart attacks were likely to have poor oral health. That was significant to them, because they were looking for a smoking gun. The risk factors they knew of for heart disease—high blood pressure, high cholesterol, type 2 diabetes and smoking—accounted for only 50 percent of heart attacks. We'll tell you more in Chapter 11, Heart Disease.

Since then, study after study has shown links, some alarmingly strong, between gum disease and the Top 5 Killers, as well as a host of other chronic preventable diseases. And those relationships are significant, even if they're not strictly cause-and-effect.

What do we mean by that? Let us give you a familiar example.

Smoking is linked to a variety of ill effects, including lung cancer. Yet some people who smoke don't get lung cancer, and some people who get lung cancer never smoked. This isn't a direct cause-and effect relationship, but there's no doubt that if you smoke, you have a greater risk of getting lung cancer and almost every other type of cancer too.

That's the same relationship periodontal disease has with many chronic diseases. We can't say that you'll get heart disease if you have gum disease—but research shows it's a major risk factor.

In this section, we'll take a look at the Top 5 Killers—heart disease, as we already mentioned, plus in Chapter 12, Cancer; Chapter 13, Stroke; Chapter 14, Diabetes; and Chapter 15, Respiratory Disease. You'll learn about how they happen, their impact, what role oral health plays and the evidence that links oral health to them. And most importantly, we also list key steps you can take to prevent them from destroying your life.

Chapter 11

HEART DISEASE: KILLER #1

IF YOU ASK ADULTS ABOUT THE LEADING CAUSE OF DEATH for women in the United States, most would say it's breast cancer. We've all been touched in some way by breast cancer and public awareness has grown to a new high. But in reality, only one in 25 women will eventually die of breast cancer. Compare that with the one in two women who will succumb to heart disease, according to the American Heart Association.

Heart disease remains the #1 killer of men and women across ethnicities and socioeconomic classes, across cultures and countries. And it's what made a 1989 study by a Finnish cardiologist attract so much attention.

Kimmo Mattila and his colleagues had noticed the poor oral health of patients admitted to the emergency room with heart attacks. So they examined the patients to evaluate their oral health. The result: Patients who had experienced heart attacks had significantly worse dental health. Even after the researchers adjusted for age, social class, smoking, cholesterol concentrations and diabetes, the link was valid.

But why did Mattila and his colleagues care what their patients' teeth and gums looked like? Because they were looking for additional risk factors for heart attacks. The traditional factors—high blood pressure and cholesterol, diabetes and smoking—explain only one in two heart attacks.

Could oral disease be a significant risk factor?

The impact of heart disease

Given that it's the #1 killer in the United States and worldwide, we need every advantage to reduce the incidence of death and decline from heart disease.

In the journal *Circulation*, the American Heart Association reported that despite decreases in the number of deaths from Cardiovascular disease (CVD)—that's heart disease and stroke combined—from 2000 to 2010, it still accounts for one of every three deaths in the United States. On average, one American dies of CVD every 40 seconds.

Heart disease alone causes one in six deaths. Every 34 seconds, an American has a coronary; every 93 seconds, an American dies from one. That adds up to 620,000 Americans who have a new heart attack each year and 295,000 more who have a recurrent attack. Despite improved survival rates, about 25 percent of men and 33 percent of women will die within a year of a first heart attack.

The World Heart Federation estimates 17.3 million people throughout the world die of CVD each year, 7.2 million of them from heart attacks.

How heart disease happens

CVD includes heart attacks, heart arrhythmia, heart valve problems and stroke. We'll address the latter in Chapter 13, Stroke, but for now we'll focus on heart attacks.

Heart attacks are usually caused from coronary artery disease (CAD)—a narrowing of your artery walls that restricts or obstructs blood flow to the heart muscle. The muscle needs the oxygen in the blood to survive, so either a little or a lot of the muscle dies.

What blocks the arteries? We hear so much about cholesterol that you might think the buildup of plaque in artery walls eventually cuts off the blood flow, triggering a heart attack.

But that's not what happens. Instead, plaque penetrates the blood vessel lining and builds up inside the walls of the artery, thickening and sometimes hardening it. In fact, we used to call this "hardening of the arteries." When the walls get too fat and the tube gets too thin, a small blood clot interferes with or blocks the blood flow. That's why many people with CAD take medication that lets the blood get through narrow spots without the risk of clotting.

There's more to the story, however. In Chapter 9, Inflammation, we discussed how chronic system inflammation (CSI) can harm otherwise healthy tissue— particularly the inner lining of our blood vessels, which is known as the endothelium. CSI can occur for a host of reasons, ranging from a long-lasting gum infection to obstructive sleep apnea to insulin resistance from ongoing sugar exposure.

You might not worry much about your endothelium until you realize that if you flattened out the lining of all your blood vessels, it would cover six tennis courts, as Bradley Bale and Amy Doneen note in their book *Beat the Heart Attack Gene*. Inflamed walls are weak walls, which make it easier for white blood cells, bad cholesterol (LDL) or even dangerous oral bacteria to penetrate them.

Once inside, bacteria multiply and form a plaque of their own. Like a pimple on your face, this plaque on the artery wall may grow and eventually rupture. The artery lining will tear soon after and the body will fix the tear with a blood clot. But if the clot is large enough to block the blood flow to the artery, you have a heart attack.

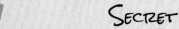

SECRET

The chance that bacterial plaque will form inside an artery wall, rupture and cause a heart attack is less about how narrow your arteries are and more about how inflamed they are. Reducing chronic inflammation in your body, including oral infection, could save your life.

The role of oral health

How does periodontal disease contribute to the sequence of events above? Researchers have proposed three primary mechanisms:

1. Chronic inflammation from gum disease: As we mentioned, periodontal disease can cause inflammation in your artery walls. Physicians use C-reactive protein (CRP), a blood marker for inflammation, to predict cardiovascular outcomes and risks. In case-control studies, people with gum disease showed a concentration of CRP that was 1.65-mg/L higher than in patients without gum disease. If your CRP is elevated, ask your dentist to evaluate you for the possibility of gum disease.

2. Traveling bacteria from gum disease: If your gums are infected, you have microbreaks in the wet skin of your mouth. Bacteria, including some dangerous species, can enter through these breaks. Although scientists once thought this occurred mainly during dental procedures, today they realize that it's probably more common during everyday activities like chewing food or brushing your teeth. Most of the bacteria get cleared by the body's natural immune system. But some bacteria enter the bloodstream and travel to new sites. They may burrow through injured arterial walls and form a plaque. As we noted, if the plaque ruptures, the blood clot that forms can block the artery and lead to heart attack or stroke.

The dental profession has focused on gum disease as a risk factor for heart disease and stroke. But there's one other mechanism that needs to be considered.

3. Traveling bacteria from tooth decay: New evidence suggests that tooth decay may also play a role in driving heart attacks. The oral bacteria species that cause tooth decay invade the tooth, as we describe in Chapter 5, Tooth

Decay. If they're not interrupted, the bacteria will invade the pulp, the nerve and blood vessel that form the living part of the tooth. That may require a root canal.

But the bacterial infection can spread from the pulp, through the root tip into the surrounding jawbone. That's called a periapical abscess. You may not know it's there because it isn't always painful, but your dentist can often spot it on an x-ray. From the abscess, the bacteria may also travel to other sites, including to and through inflamed walls of your arteries, to form plaques.

SECRET

The interleukin-1 saliva test can help identify your genetic risk for both coronary artery disease and periodontal disease. If you test positive, it is crucial that you maintain good lifestyle choices and oral healthcare, including professional cleanings every three months, to reduce your risk of heart attack and stroke.

Evidence of a link

To clarify the link between cardiovascular disease and periodontitis, heart disease and gum disease experts reviewed more than 120 published medical studies, position papers and other data. They developed a consensus report, published simultaneously in 2009 in the *Journal of Periodontology* and the *American Journal of Cardiology*. The report confirms that studies find gum disease is a risk factor for coronary artery disease.

What about the evidence that tooth decay may play a role? A study led by Dr. Tanja Pessi and reported in the American Heart Association's journal *Circulation* demonstrated that endodontic disease is also a significant player in driving heart attack. DNA analysis of the bacteria in 101 arterial blood clots showed that 75 percent of the clots contained oral bacteria that cause cavities and 35 percent had bacteria that cause gum disease.

> ## Secret
>
> The bacteria that cause cavities can also travel. To reduce your risk of heart attack and stroke, getting cavities filled and decay under control may be just as important as addressing periodontal disease.

If you find signs of oral disease, from active decay to bleeding, red or puffy gums—or if you're putting off treatment your dentist recommends—think again. You need to act to avoid a possible risk of heart attack and stroke, as well as other serious diseases. Healthy gums and bone support are critical to keep your teeth for a lifetime, and they may save your life.

Quickstart to prevent heart disease

1. Brush, floss and get gum disease treated.

The goal is to continually reduce the bacterial load and inflammation in your mouth.

2. Address and control tooth decay.

Cavity-causing bacteria can create an abscess and increase your risk of heart disease. So if you have cavities, get them filled. If you don't, make a plan to keep it that way.

3. Get an interleukin-1 saliva test from your dentist.

If your dentist does not offer this test routinely, request that he order it through a genetics diagnostic lab, such as Oral DNA Labs. If your result is positive, you will need to discuss a personalized plan to prevent coronary artery disease with your physician. You'll also have a hyper-inflammatory response to dangerous oral bacteria, which will put you at risk for faster progression of gum infection, bone loss and ultimately tooth loss. Be diligent about home care and see your dentist for a thorough professional cleaning every three months.

4. Don't smoke.

Smoking is a huge risk factor for heart disease and also for a hundred other chronic diseases. If you smoke, quit; if you don't smoke, don't start. Learn more in Chapter 42, Cigarettes and Chew.

5. Eat an anti-inflammatory diet.

To combat inflammation, improve the quality of your foods, shifting from processed to whole foods. Reduce your sugar consumption and eliminate hydrogenated, saturated and trans fats. Load up on fresh fruits and vegetables. And limit salt, because it can increase your blood pressure.

6. Exercise daily.

Sitting shows up in a variety of ways: excess weight, high blood pressure and high blood sugar, to name a few. These all increase risk of CVD. If you hate exercise, think of one activity you like that requires movement and commit to doing it for just 10 minutes a day. Those 10 minutes often lead to more—and the more fit you get, the more you will enjoy it.

7. Limit alcohol.

Too much alcohol can be bad news for your overall health. But because it raises your blood pressure, excessive alcohol can be particularly bad for heart disease. Limit consumption to two drinks a day if you're a man and one drink a day if you're a woman. Learn more in Chapter 41, Alcohol.

8. Inform your physician and your dentist of all your known risk factors for CVD.

Working together, they'll be able to develop a treatment plan personalized for you. So make sure they both know about active gum disease, cavities, high blood pressure, smoking, insulin resistance or a family history of CVD. As a team, they can help you to improve your oral health and reduce your heart disease risk.

Blabber M●uth!

Chapter 12

CANCER: KILLER #2

IN CHAPTER 27, WE'LL COVER THE LATEST INFORMATION on Oral Cancer. But we'll mention it here first, because one of the earliest studies linking oral health and a chronic disease involved oral cancer.

Back in 1957, three researchers from Sloan-Kettering Institute for Cancer Research and the Cornell University Medical College took a look at factors that cause oral cancer to develop. In addition to the usual suspects, such as tobacco use, alcohol consumption, nutritional deficiencies and sunlight exposure, they included oral trauma, infection and dental irritation.

Not surprisingly, tobacco and alcohol were found to be significant causes; trauma and dental irritation were not. But the researchers did note that losing all your teeth—the unhappy circumstance known as *edentulism*—was more common among mouth-cancer patients, particularly women. It was a clue that oral infection might be a factor after all.

Fast forward a few decades to the late 1980s, when Finnish researchers made the connection between heart attacks and poor oral health. Since then, numerous studies have shown links between gum disease and serious systemic diseases, including heart disease, diabetes, pregnancy complications and osteoporosis.

So it's no surprise that researchers reopened the case for a link between periodontitis and cancers of all kinds. Another compelling factor was the World Health Organization's designation of three common mouth dwellers as human carcinogens: *Helicobacter pylori*, commonly associated with stomach ulcers, and both the human papillomavirus (HPV) and Epstein-Barr virus (the one that causes mononucleosis).

In this chapter, we'll look at associations between periodontitis and cancer of the mouth, lung and pancreas.

Impact of cancer

Killer #2, cancer, causes the deaths of one in four Americans. The American Cancer Society estimated that in 2015, 1,658,370 people in the United States would be diagnosed with some form of cancer and 589,430 would die of it—more than one person every minute.

Worldwide, WHO predicted approximately 14 million new cases of cancer and 8.2 million deaths from the disease in 2012. Over the next two decades, the number of new cases is expected to increase by about 70 percent.

And yet, cancer is not inevitable. You can often prevent cancer or reduce the risk of it through lifestyle changes. Those changes including eating a nutritious diet, eliminating tobacco, drinking alcohol in moderation, exercising regularly and using vaccinations/antibiotics against viruses and bacteria.

How cancer happens

To better understand cancer's association with periodontal disease, let's quickly review how it develops. In health, the body's cells grow, divide to create new cells and then die, just like clockwork. If you've watched how fast children grow, you know their cells are going through this process must faster than the cells of their grandparents.

But cancer cells are mutations of the original cells that have gone awry. They don't die a normal death. Instead they grow faster than normal, crowding out the healthy cells around them. They also have other unique and unfortunate capabilities—they can invade tissues and even travel to other parts of the body. In the process called metastasis, they form new tumors far from their original home.

All body cells, including cancer cells, have DNA to direct their growth, repair and death. In cancer cells, however, the DNA is damaged. You can inherit abnormal DNA, but it can also occur as a traumatic incident when a normal cell is dividing or when something in the environment triggers damage. That something could be cigarette smoke or alcohol use or a virus.

A virus is a very small organism that enters a cell, injects its own DNA and hijacks the cell's machinery to make more viruses. But the virus' DNA can also alter the host cell's DNA and push it toward cancer. The most relevant to oral health is human papillomavirus (HPV), which can lead to both cervical and oral cancer, as we discuss in Chapter 27, Oral Cancer.

The role of oral health

As we mentioned above, some of the catalysts for cancer include injury, infection and your inflammatory response to infection.

So you may have guessed that periodontitis would be associated with cancer. In a healthy mouth, billions of bacteria live and play happily together in a large community. But in the right environment—often one in which oral hygiene isn't up to par—bad bacteria gain a foothold and start taking over.

That produces an infection, which triggers inflammation as well. Certain dangerous bacteria can spread beyond the gums to other parts of your body— easily to the lungs and digestive tract, but even to locations far beyond via the bloodstream. The byproducts of inflammation also circulate throughout your body and create their own insult, which causes cell damage.

Evidence of a link

Many studies have looked at the link between oral health, specifically periodontitis, and cancer. But a caveat here: The studies use many different measures of oral health, from oral condition (such things as tooth brushing, hygiene and restorations) to tooth loss and periodontal disease. The strongest evidence links cancer with periodontal disease—but as you might imagine, it's challenging for researchers to conduct hands-on periodontal assessments of the subjects in a research study. Instead they use proxies like tooth loss—which could be the result of periodontal disease or of trauma, tooth decay or other causes.

One study in *Lancet Oncology* reported the work of cancer epidemiologist Dominique Michaud and colleagues, who surveyed more than 48,000 American health professionals. After 18 years of follow-up, 5,720 cases of cancer were reported. After adjusting for risk factors such as smoking and diet, the researchers found that individuals with periodontal disease had a 14 percent higher risk of developing some kind of cancer. Specific types of cancer had higher risks: 36 percent for lung cancer, 49 percent for kidney cancer, 54 percent for pancreatic cancer, and 30 percent for white blood cell cancers.

Let's look closer below for connections between several types of cancer and oral health.

Oral cancer

The American Cancer Society estimates that in 2015, about 39,500 people will be diagnosed with mouth or oropharyngeal cancer, and 7,500 people will die of these cancers.

But the real news is the startling rise in oral cancers—and the cause. Although the incidence of many other cancers is declining, oral cancer has increased each of the last six years—and it's the cancer that's growing fastest among young non-smokers. At the present time, it's estimated that approximately 60 percent of cancers of the mouth are caused by HPV.

But does your risk of oral cancer increase if you have gum disease?

To answer that question, a research team conducted a study between 1999 and 2005 at the Rosewell Park Cancer Institute in New York. The study showed a direct association between chronic gum disease and tongue cancer, even after adjusting for factors such as smoking status, age and gender. Each tiny millimeter of tooth-supporting bone loss increased the risk of tongue cancer more than five times.

Another group of researchers took a look at the big picture by reviewing select PubMed articles from 1995 to 2010 that discussed the possible role of tooth loss and periodontal disease in cancer. Nine of 10 case-control studies reported a significant increase in the risk of oral cancer in patients with periodontitis.

So is there a link between severe periodontal disease and oral cancer? Based on research to date, it appears a link exists, even after adjusting research results for smoking and drinking.

Lung cancer

The American Cancer Society projected that 221,200 Americans would be diagnosed with lung cancer in 2015 and 158,040 would die from it. Lung cancer is the second most common cancer for all adults, behind prostate cancer in men and breast cancer in women. With that high an incidence, researchers will look at any possible way to reduce risk.

In a study reported in 2003, investigators used data from the National Health and Nutrition Examination Survey I (NHANES I) to investigate the link between periodontitis and various cancers, including lung cancer. Gum disease proved to be the strongest association found. After adjusting for known lung cancer risk factors such as smoking, the study found the increased risk of dying from lung cancer ranged from 48 percent to 73 percent for those with periodontitis.

In the survey of U.S. health professionals reported by Michaud and colleagues in 2008, fewer teeth at the start of the study (0-16) was associated with a 70 percent increased risk of getting lung cancer, as compared to those with 25-32 teeth. In those who never smoked, however, the researchers found no association for lung cancer.

A study conducted in Scotland in 2007 also found no significant association between tooth loss and death from lung cancer, even with adjustment for smoking status.

At this point, the confounding factor of smoking makes it tricky to determine the role of periodontal disease alone in the development of lung cancer. We need further studies to tease out the relationship.

Pancreatic cancer

Pancreatic cancer is the fourth leading cause of cancer death in the United States. The diagnosis is devastating, because the disease is so difficult to treat. The American Cancer Society estimates 48,960 new cases of pancreatic cancer in 2015 and 40,560 deaths.

In the NHANES study mentioned above, Hujoel and colleagues confirmed an increased risk for pancreatic cancer among subjects with periodontitis.

Research by Harvard's Dominique Michaud looked at U.S. and then European male health professionals and found a significant association between periodontal disease and pancreatic cancer. The 2007 study was one of the first to control for smoking, a factor in both diseases. Overall, the relative risk of pancreatic cancer increased 64 percent in study subjects with periodontitis.

In an intriguing 2012 study of individuals with pancreatic cancer and controls in Europe, the researchers measured levels of antibodies to 25 specific oral bacteria. They identified higher levels of antibodies specific to bacteria most often present in periodontal disease. For example, people with high levels of antibodies to *Porphyromonas gingivalis* had more than twice the risk of pancreatic cancer than did those with low levels.

The good news is that high levels of antibodies to oral bacteria not associated with periodontitis—the "good" bacteria in your mouth—appeared to be protective against pancreatic cancer.

Quickstart to prevent cancer

1. Screen for all the pre-cancerous growths you can.

Pap smears and colonoscopies screen pre-cancerous cells in the cervix and colon. Mammograms help find early, often highly treatable, breast cancer. And removing dark, asymmetric moles can sometimes remove melanoma before it's lethal. Oral cancer screenings in your dental office can help identify suspicious areas to be biopsied. Better yet, ask your dentist to test your saliva for persistent HPV infection, which poses the greatest risk for oral cancer. Also ask about a high-tech illumination instrument for pre-cancer detection.

2. Avoid smoking or chewing tobacco.

The most important risk factor for cancer is tobacco, which causes more than 20 percent of cancer deaths globally and about 70 percent of lung cancer deaths worldwide. If you don't use, don't start, and if you do, quit. Learn more in Chapter 42, Cigarettes and Chew.

3. Drink alcohol in moderation.

Drinking alcohol has been linked to cancers of the mouth, throat, voice box, esophagus, liver, colon and breast. The risk increases with the amount of alcohol consumed. Limit alcohol to two drinks a day for men and one drink a day for women. Learn more in Chapter 41, Alcohol.

4. Maintain a healthy weight, eat a diet rich in fruits and vegetables, and exercise five days each week.

The World Cancer Research Fund estimates that one-third of cancer cases in economically developed countries like the United States are related to excess weight, poor nutrition and a sedentary lifestyle.

5. Protect skin from ultraviolet rays.

Many cases of skin cancer (basal cell, squamous cell and melanoma) as well as squamous cell cancer of the lower lip can be prevented by using sunscreen with an SPF of at least 15 when outdoors. Also avoid indoor tanning.

Chapter 13

STROKE: KILLER #3

From the chair

As a young man, Pete was a regular patient, a strapping construction worker with his own stamping concrete business. But for a decade, he stopped visiting our dental office. When he returned at the age of 44, we barely recognized him. He walked with a limp, dragging his left foot. His left hand was almost useless.

At only 43, Pete suffered a paralyzing stroke. He'd had a restless night's sleep, flopped out of bed and couldn't get up. His wife called an ambulance.

After a month in the hospital and seven months of diligent work in rehab, Pete leads an independent life—but with the risk of another stroke clouding his future. Why? Because none of Pete's doctors, including his vascular neurologist—the stroke doctor—could identify any risk factors. There was nothing they could fix. Pete did not have high blood pressure, excess body fat or a family history of stroke, and he didn't smoke, drink or use drugs.

During his 10-year hiatus from our practice, Pete brushed his teeth hurriedly in the morning and before bed, but he never flossed. He stayed away because "nothing hurt." When he finally returned to get his teeth cleaned, he had full-blown periodontal disease—a known risk factor for stroke that not one of his physicians had ever mentioned. The news was actually a relief to Pete as well as to his mom, who had worked tirelessly to discover any possible unknown factors that might keep her boy at risk for another stroke, one that might this time take his life.

Pete gladly accepted gum disease treatment. Just like with his stroke rehab, he became the champion of his disease. He now spends a solid 8 to 10 minutes a day carefully following his new protocol: spin brushing, deep flossing, rinsing with a water jet and, every three months, professional periodontal cleanings, readdressing any little area of inflammation that crops up.

The impact of stroke

Stroke is the #3 killer in the United States, exceeded only by heart disease and cancer, according to the Centers for Disease Control and Prevention. But if you had asked Dr. Susan's dad, who suffered six strokes within seven years, what's perhaps worse than dying from a stroke? He'd have said it's living with the crippling loss of body function and dependence on others for almost every aspect of his life.

Every 40 seconds an American suffers a stroke and every four minutes someone dies from a stroke, according to the American Heart Association (AHA). That adds up to 795,000 Americans who experience a stroke every year, 610,000 for the first time.

Worldwide 15 million people suffer a stroke annually. Some 3 million women and 2.5 million men die of stroke each year. That's right: Women have a higher lifetime risk of stroke than men, even adjusting for age.

That's a lot of numbers and still doesn't paint the whole picture. Even if, like Pete and Susan's dad, you beat death, stroke can result in paralysis, loss of vision and/or speech and brain dysfunction. The World Health Organization estimates that 5 million people worldwide are left permanently disabled each year after a stroke.

Stroke costs the United States an estimated $36.5 billion each year, including the cost of healthcare services, medications to treat stroke and missed days of work. And that cost will rise. Currently an estimated 6.8 million Americans age 20 or over have had a stroke. But by 2030, the AHA projects an additional 3.4 million people age 18 and over will be victims.

How stroke happens

We covered the basics of cardiovascular disease in Chapter 11, Heart Disease.

You can think of stroke as a brain attack versus a heart attack. For your brain to work, it needs blood. If the blood stops flowing due to a blockage—a narrowing or bursting blood vessel or a blood clot moving to the brain—the brain loses its lifeline. When any part of the brain is deprived of oxygen and nutrients, it dies, and with it goes the body function it handled.

The overwhelming majority of strokes (87 percent) are *ischemic*—due to an obstruction within a blood vessel supplying blood to the brain. You've probably heard of *transient ischemic attacks* or TIAs, which are caused by a temporary clot, but are still serious. More serious still are the 10 percent of strokes classified as *hemorrhagic*, which occur when a weakened blood vessel breaks open.

The most common cause of stroke is uncontrolled high blood pressure, an often silent condition that directly stresses the blood vessels.

The role of oral health

In 1986, Syrjanen and his colleagues suggested that chronic inflammation could be a risk factor for stroke. Periodontitis is one of the most common causes of inflammation in the body.

But stroke and periodontitis share many risk factors—age, smoking, high blood pressure, diabetes, cardiovascular disease, physical inactivity and poor nutrition. So we need to tease out why there might be an association between periodontitis and stroke beyond these factors.

Researchers have proposed the two main mechanisms we cover in Section 3: The Chronic Connection. For more detail, take a look at Chapter 9, Inflammation, and Chapter 10, Traveling Bacteria.

Evidence of a link

A number of studies have shown a correlation between periodontitis or missing teeth and stroke. For example, Wu and colleagues reported in 2000 on how periodontitis might contribute to stroke risk using data from the National Health and Nutrition Evaluation Survey I population of 9,962 individuals. The investigators reported that clinical periodontitis increased the risk for fatal and nonfatal strokes slightly more than twofold.

Case-control studies also report that the concentration of the inflammation marker CRP (C-reactive protein) is significantly greater in individuals with gum disease compared to those without the disease. CRP is used to predict cardiovascular outcomes and risks.

In April 2012, a team of physicians in Greece reviewed the relationship between periodontal disease and stroke in published studies. After whittling down the 146 original studies to 13 that met their criteria—for example, studies on humans, not animals—they looked at the association between periodontitis and stroke.

Patients in the studies had suffered both ischemic and hemorrhagic strokes. Most controlled for risk factors that periodontitis and stroke have in common.

The researchers concluded there is evidence that periodontitis is associated with increased risk of stroke. Overall adjusted risk of stroke in patients with periodontitis was 1.47 times to 2.63 times higher. Even when the results were adjusted for publication bias—in other words, for the fact that people generally don't publish studies in which they find nothing—the results still indicated an association.

For now, you can help prevent stroke by following the steps below. They may sound similar to those for heart disease, but consider that a bonus—preventing two diseases instead of one.

Quickstart to prevent stroke

1. Get gum disease treated.

Get regular periodontal exams and have all gum disease treated to reduce the bacterial load and inflammation in your mouth. If you have a history of gum disease or bone loss that leaves you with hard-to-reach areas that harbor bacteria, get your teeth professionally cleaned every three months.

2. Tell your physician and dentist about all your risk factors for stroke, including gum disease.

If you have high blood pressure, particularly if it's untreated, see your dentist. If you have gum disease, tell your physician. If you have another risk factor too, such as high blood pressure or smoking, tell all your docs. Working together they'll be able to develop a treatment plan personalized for you.

3. Get an interleukin-1 saliva test from your dentist.

Your dentist may not offer this test routinely, but she can order it through a genetics diagnostic lab. A single genetic test measures the risk levels of both gum disease and cardiovascular disease. If you test positive, you need to discuss a personalized prevention plan with your dentist and your physician.

4. Keep your blood pressure under control.

The #1 risk factor for stroke is high blood pressure. High blood pressure has no symptoms, so make sure you check yours on a regular basis. If you take medication for high blood pressure, be sure to take it as prescribed.

BlabberM⬤uth!

5. Eat a healthy diet.

By healthy, we mean a diet that puts your body in an optimal state of healing and keeps your cholesterol under control. Eat foods low in sugar, saturated fats, trans fat and hydrogenated fats. Load up on fresh fruits and vegetables. And to further reduce your risk of high blood pressure, limit sodium intake including table salt, canned foods, processed foods and soda, which is loaded with salt.

6. Get 2½ hours of exercise each week.

The good news is that exercise can help you lower your blood pressure, increase your "good" cholesterol and maintain a healthy weight. Five days a week, you should get at least half an hour of moderate intensity exercise—like walking briskly or bicycling.

7. Don't smoke.

Quitting tobacco use will reduce your risk of stroke—and so many other diseases that we can't begin to list them all. Learn more in Chapter 42, Cigarettes and Chew.

8. Limit alcohol.

Too much alcohol can be bad news for your overall health, but it's particularly bad for stroke, because it can raise your blood pressure. Limit drinks to two per day if you're a man and one per day if you're a woman. Learn more in Chapter 41, Alcohol.

Chapter 14

DIABETES: KILLER #4

From the chair

ANNA HAD WORKED AS MY DENTAL ASSISTANT *for several years before her 33-year-old baby sister, Andréa, asked for an appointment with me. Andréa's front teeth were drifting apart, making her self-conscious about her smile. She wanted braces.*

After x-rays and a dental exam, it was obvious that braces wouldn't solve the problem. Andréa's teeth were moving because she was rapidly losing bone support. She had full-blown gum disease even though she brushed and flossed twice a day and didn't smoke.

I immediately suspected that diabetes was causing her aggressive gum disease. Although Andréa's health history was pretty clean, she had two obvious risk factors for diabetes—she was significantly overweight and Hispanic-American.

On the Diabetes Self-Screen you'll see later in this chapter, Andréa scored moderate- to high-risk. She also disclosed that she had recently lost 15 pounds, almost without trying. I ordered an A1c blood test to measure her 3-month average blood glucose level. The results? Sky high at 14.

Anna knew several family members had been diagnosed with diabetes, a disease that can turn the life-giving blood in your veins into a corrosive liquid. The sisters' maternal grandmother had passed away from complications of the disease.

One year later, Andréa has lost more than 90 pounds and lowered her blood glucose level to 8. It's still too high, but she's working hard. She stopped drinking soda and alcohol, cut down on junk-carb foods and exercises at least three times a week. She is under a physician's care and taking prescription medication to help lower her blood sugar.

And of critical importance, we're aggressively treating Andréa's gum disease, because without stability it's really hard to control her blood sugar—and vice versa. Diabetic patients like Andrea begin to suffer from gum disease at an earlier age, have more severe infection and bone loss, and don't heal as well in response to traditional therapy.

The impact of diabetes

Type 2 diabetes is now an epidemic, with increasing health and financial burdens in the United States and worldwide. Diabetes and its precursor, prediabetes, together affect 103 million people, one-third of the U.S. population. But about 28 percent of patients with diabetes and 93 percent of those with prediabetes don't know it. By the year 2050, one in three of us are projected to be diabetic.

Maybe you've heard that diabetes is the leading cause of new cases of blindness and of kidney failure, or that more than 60 percent of lower limbs amputated in non-trauma cases are due to diabetes. But did you know that diabetics have death rates due to heart disease and stroke that are two to four times that of people without the disease? Also realize that if you become diabetic, you'll likely suffer from nervous system damage as well as increased rates of dementia and Alzheimer's disease.

Currently 29 million Americans are diabetic but about 8 million don't know it yet. We spend more than $300 billion annually to care for the almost 21 million known diabetics. That's more than 20 percent of our total healthcare expenditure. But given the projections that more than 100 million Americans will become diabetics, the costs for treatment will cripple the U.S. healthcare system.

There's one more statistic that you may not be aware of: After analyzing the data from the National Health and Nutrition Examination Survey for 2009-2010, researchers found that a startling 60 percent of those with diabetes had moderate to severe periodontal disease.

How diabetes happens

Most people know that type 2 diabetes stems from problems controlling blood sugar—which is primarily a cascading effect from over-exposure to sugar itself. For thousands of years, the only sugar humans ate was packed into fruits and vegetables, and came with an antidote to slow down uptake—fiber. The only form of straight-up sugar was honey, which was well-protected by bees. But as you know, today we take sugar from sugar cane, beets and corn and tuck it into hundreds of foods. We'll tell you more about America's out-of-control sugar consumption in Chapter 43, Sugar.

For now, you need to know that our bodies do one of two things with sugar:

• use it as an immediate energy source; or

• store it for another time, often as fat.

It's not just fat storage that hurts us, however; it's the system breakdown that occurs along the way. When we eat or drink foods with refined sugar, we get an immediate blood-sugar rush, which triggers an insulin spike. Insulin tells the cells in the liver, muscle and fat tissue to take up glucose—sugar—from the blood and store it.

If you constantly bombard your body with sugar, your cells become resistant to the constant outpouring of insulin. This condition is known as *insulin resistance*, and it's an inflammatory pre-diabetic condition. Keep up the sugar intake and your pancreas' insulin pump eventually burns out. Now you have too much free sugar in the bloodstream, which damages your blood vessels.

The fat that makes our jeans too tight is reflected inside the body by fat that accumulates around and within vital organs. One example is fatty liver disease—the nonalcoholic version of the disease that can lead to cirrhosis of the liver, liver cancer or liver failure. That triggers the production of bad cholesterol, increasing your risk of cardiovascular disease.

Keep in mind that by the time diabetes is diagnosed, significant complications have already occurred. In fact, one researcher estimated that at least 10 years *of potential preventive measures* are wasted before diabetes is diagnosed.

The role of oral health

As we said above, gum disease complicates blood sugar control—and diabetes complicates gum disease treatment. The effects of periodontitis and diabetes on each other are likely due to the fact that both contribute to a hyper-inflammatory state in the body.

Dr. Susan asserts that managing gum disease for the unidentified diabetic is like trying to wrestle a gorilla with one hand tied behind her back. It's hard enough with two hands.

For this reason. Dr. Susan wanted to routinely screen her patients for diabetes. But all the validated screening surveys, like the one on the American Diabetes Association website, seemed to include BMI, which requires weighing a patient.

You've probably never been weighed at the dental office and that probably isn't going to change soon. So Dr. Susan partnered with Dr. Saleh Aldasouqi, chairman of Michigan State University's Division of Endocrinology, to conduct research on diabetes and prediabetes screening. The project was called "DiDDO: Diabetes Detection in the Dental Office."

Dr. Susan randomly tested 500 of her adult patients' blood sugar levels with an A1c fingerstick blood test. The same patients answered a 14-question proposed risk assessment for diabetes and the blood results were statistically compared to their answers. What's unique in the DiDDO survey is that none of the questions asked for body weight or BMI, *or* required clinical data such as blood pressure or blood lipid level measurements. The result is the following validated, dental-office-friendly self-screening tool.

Your risk of diabetes

To determine if you're at risk for diabetes, you can start with an assessment using Dr. Susan's self-screening tool. To take the test on your smart phone or tablet, or to share it with others, just go to http://SelfScreen.net or use the QR code below.

Diabetes Risk Assessment

Scoring: Yes=1 point, No=0 points

_____ Are you more than 10 percent above ideal body weight OR is your waist above 35" for women or 40" for men?

_____ Do you have any biologic family member with a history of diabetes?

_____ Are you of African American, Alaskan Native, American Indian, Hispanic, or Arabic descent?

_____ Do you have a history of or take medication for high blood pressure?

_____ Do you have or take medications for high cholesterol or abnormal good/bad cholesterol ratio?

_____ Do you experience tingling, pain or numbness in your hands or feet?

_____ Do you experience unexplainable hunger, thirst or frequent urination?

_____ Have you experienced blurred vision, cataracts or glaucoma?

_____ Do your gums bleed when you brush or floss?

Age:

_____ Are you over 35?

_____ If you are over 35, are you also over 65?

_____ **Total points**

Score total points:

0-2 Low risk for prediabetes and diabetes: Learn more about prevention

3+ Moderate to high risk: Get further diagnostic testing for prediabetes and diabetes

BlabberM😮uth!

If you are at moderate to high risk for prediabetes or diabetes, how do you get a diagnosis? The available blood tests are A1c, FPG (fasting plasma glucose) and OGTT (oral glucose tolerance test). The American Diabetes Association recommends the A1c test, mostly because it does not require fasting.

Approval is pending with the Food and Drug Administration for A1c to be used for point-of-care diagnosis using a highly accurate, affordable, countertop photometer that needs only one drop of blood for a diagnosis. Soon you can expect that your dental office will be able to diagnose diabetes right on the spot.

Evidence of a link

Multiple studies have shown that early onset or rapidly progressing periodontal disease that either starts when a patient is still young, progresses rapidly or fails to respond to traditional periodontal therapy can be indicators of poor blood sugar control in the diabetic patient. In fact, researchers studying the relationship between periodontal disease and diabetes in German patients found that diabetes control was associated with future tooth loss and faster progression of bone loss.

Several systematic reviews have also shown that active periodontal infection adversely influences the diabetic patient's ability to achieve blood sugar control. And one significant study by Javed and colleagues reported that even moderately high blood sugar—at the levels seen in prediabetes—can be enough to trigger periodontal disease.

Although periodontal disease may prove to be an independent risk factor for type 2 diabetes, further research must be done to determine if treating periodontal disease will reduce the onset or progression of diabetes and the burden of disease complications.

Quickstart to prevent diabetes

1. Get screened for diabetes.

Take the risk assessment above. If your score places you at moderate or high risk, get a diagnostic blood test. Diabetes is nothing to be casual about—if you have it, or even prediabetes, it can take years off your life.

2. Treat periodontal disease.

If you have untreated gum disease, talk to your dentist about getting it treated. That's especially important if you've been diagnosed with prediabetes or diabetes.

3. Eat a low-sugar, high-fiber diet.

If you have diabetes or prediabetes, your diet is critical to controlling your blood sugar, lipids and weight. Focus on lean protein, whole grains, fruits, vegetables and low-fat milk. Increase your fiber to stave off insulin spikes and restrict the intake of refined carbs and sweets, including sweetened beverages.

4. Exercise.

Exercise can immediately reduce high blood sugar levels. Over time it can help you lose weight and increase insulin sensitivity, which may both halt the progression of diabetes.

5. Lose weight.

You can be thin and diabetic, but if you are overweight and you lose weight, you may halt the progression of diabetes. One study showed that losing 7 to 10 percent of body weight and exercising five times a week for 30 minutes reduced the incidence of type 2 diabetes by 58 percent over three years, compared to a control group that didn't make lifestyle changes.

6. Work with your physician and dentist.

If you have diabetes, know your blood sugar numbers. Due to the strong association between uncontrolled blood sugar and periodontal disease, you need to work closely with both your dentist and physician to manage diabetes.

Chapter 15

RESPIRATORY DISEASE: KILLER #5

He played an alien—or half of one—so logical, yet so lovable, that humans around the globe worshipped him. As the first officer of the Starship Enterprise, Leonard Nimoy helped propel the television show and movie *Star Trek* to juggernaut status. As late as 2013, Nimoy stepped into the iconic role of Mr. Spock, playing a much older version of the Vulcan who'd first arrived in homes across America in the 1960s. But in February 2015, at the age of 83, he passed on of *chronic obstructive pulmonary disorder* (COPD).

You've probably seen the abbreviation COPD before, but what is it? The disease has a variety of guises, but the main abnormality is airflow limitation that cannot be fully reversed. In fact, the limitation usually worsens over time. COPD is second only to heart disease as a cause of disability. In developed countries, COPD stands out as the major chronic disease for which deaths are on the rise.

COPD is one of several chronic respiratory diseases that affect the airways and other structures of the lungs. Although the group includes asthma, sleep apnea, lung cancer and others, we're going to focus on just two diseases in this chapter: COPD and pneumonia.

You're probably already familiar with pneumonia, which is a bacterial or viral infection of the lungs. The symptoms include cough, fever, chills and trouble breathing. The disease becomes deadly when your lungs can no longer move oxygen into the bloodstream, shutting off the supply to your body's cells. Combined with the spreading infection, this can cause death.

> ## " SECRET
>
> Respiratory infections commonly occur when secretions from the mouth and throat get sucked into the lungs. These secretions contain microorganisms, like bacteria and viruses, which can lead to COPD or pneumonia. Keeping your mouth free of oral infection can reduce your risk of illness and death from lung disease. "

The impact of respiratory disease

In the United States, about 12 million people have been diagnosed with COPD—but just as many may have the disease and not know it. In 2010, approximately 135,000 Americans died of COPD. Treating the disease costs more than $49 billion each year, mainly due to the hospital visits required as COPD worsens.

Around the globe, COPD affects 200 million people and is a major cause of disease and death, according to a study published in *Lancet*. Because physicians cannot usually diagnose COPD until clinical signs are apparent, the disease is often advanced and more difficult and expensive to treat.

The World Health Organization estimates that 4 to 20 percent of adults over 40 suffer from COPD, and the incidence increases with age, particularly among smokers. By 2030, WHO projects COPD will rank as the fourth leading cause of death worldwide.

Pneumonia also remains a serious disease, both in the United States and globally. According to the Centers for Disease Control and Prevention, more than 1.1 million Americans are hospitalized each year due to pneumonia. An additional 33,700 residents of nursing homes are stricken with pneumonia, and more than 53,000 people die of the disease annually.

Worldwide pneumonia is the #1 infectious cause of death among children, killing 15 percent of those under 5 years of age. In 2013 alone, pneumonia was responsible for the deaths of an estimated 935,000 young children.

How respiratory disease happens

So what causes COPD? Not surprisingly, the main cause is long-term smoking. In fact, Nimoy's COPD resulted from smoking. Although he'd quit 30 years before his death, the lung damage remained. One of his last tweets read, "Don't smoke. I did. Wish I never had. LLAP." (LLAP? Live long and prosper.)

About 20 percent of chronic smokers develop COPD. They also put friends and family at risk from secondhand smoke. In developing countries, women experience a particularly high incidence of COPD due to the amount of time they spend in poorly ventilated homes. There they are exposed to fumes from wood and animal wastes burned for cooking and heating. Other dangerous irritants include air pollution and workplace exposure to dust, smoke and fumes.

As we said, COPD occurs due to airway limitation—but what exactly does that mean? When you breathe in, air travels first down your windpipe, then through two large tubes known as the *bronchi*. You have two lungs, of course, and inside them the tubes divide many times in tree-like fashion into *bronchioles*—small tubes—and *alveoli*—tiny air sacs that look like bubble wrap under a microscope. The alveoli are formed by thin walls of blood vessels, which are elastic so they can stretch like a balloon when filled with air and shrink when emptied.

Breathe in and the oxygen crosses over into these blood vessels, attaches to red blood cells and enters your bloodstream. Breathe out and the flow of carbon dioxide rids your body of the waste products of metabolism.

Your lungs count on the elasticity of the tubes and sacs to enable that flow. But COPD causes the walls to become thick and inflamed, limiting their ability to stretch. Air gets trapped in your lungs, which swell and become clogged with mucus. You lose out on oxygen going in and keep too much of the carbon dioxide that's supposed to be going out. Breathing becomes hard.

In pneumonia, inflammation causes the air sacs to fill with fluid or pus, and the lungs struggle to get oxygen into the blood. The cause of the disease is usually a viral or bacterial infection, making people with weakened or compromised immune systems especially susceptible—including the elderly, smokers, alcoholics and children in underdeveloped countries.

The role of oral health

COPD and pneumonia have both been associated with poor oral health. If you have periodontitis, for example, bacteria present in the gum pockets may gain easy access to the blood vessels and travel from there to the lungs. But most common respiratory infections occur when secretions from the mouth and throat are aspirated into the lungs. Microorganisms can infect the respiratory tract, leading to COPD or pneumonia.

Bacteria from the oral cavity may also be introduced into your respiratory system during *intubation* in the hospital—placing a flexible plastic tube down your windpipe to keep the airway open or to administer drugs.

In addition, periodontitis produces inflammatory mediators, the cytokines that we discussed in Chapter 9, Inflammation. These can be aspirated and cause inflammation in the lower airway.

Evidence of a link

Many studies have shown strong evidence that poor oral health and COPD may be linked. One early study used data from the National Health and Nutrition Examination Survey I (NHANES I) on the general health status of 23,808 people. Of those, 386 reported chronic respiratory disease (either bronchitis or emphysema) or acute disease (flu, pneumonia or acute bronchitis). After controlling for gender, age and race, the researchers found that those with a respiratory illness had significantly higher measures of oral plaque and calculus. And those with acute disease tended to have more decayed teeth.

A study of male veterans concluded that periodontitis, measured as loss of bone around teeth, was an independent risk factor for COPD. At baseline, the veterans were medically healthy. But of the 1,118 with teeth, 261 later developed COPD. The researchers found that those with the worst bone loss had an 80 percent higher risk of developing COPD.

A recent study published in the *Journal of Periodontology* confirms that periodontitis may increase the risk of respiratory infections, such as COPD and pneumonia. The study included 200 subjects between the ages of 20 and 60, all with at least 20 natural teeth. Half were hospitalized with a respiratory disease; the others were healthy. Each underwent a thorough periodontal evaluation. The upshot? Patients with respiratory diseases had worse periodontal health than the control subjects.

A major concern for patients in the hospital, especially those with long-lasting lung diseases, is hospital-acquired pneumonia. Given their illnesses, these patients often become lax about oral hygiene. Dental plaque serves as a potential reservoir of harmful respiratory bugs. In fact, the teeth of patients admitted to hospitals or long-term care facilities for respiratory disorders are often colonized by bacteria known to cause pneumonia.

The prevalence of these dangerous bacteria in the mouths of hospitalized patients was confirmed in a Romanian study. Researchers studied 34 patients hospitalized with lung disease and compared them to 31 dental outpatients with healthy lungs. The researchers detected harmful respiratory bacteria in the plaque of 29 of the 34 (85.3 percent) hospitalized patients versus only 12 of the 31 (38.7 percent) control subjects.

The bottom line: The cleaner you keep your mouth, the less chance you have of breathing dangerous microorganisms into your lungs that can cause deadly infections.

LLAP.

Quickstart to prevent respiratory disease

1. Don't smoke.

This is the no-brainer, #1 way to prevent COPD or slow it down if you already have it. If you don't smoke, don't start. If you smoke, quit. Ask your dentist, physician, family, and friends to help you—support is the key to quitting for the last time. Read more in Chapter 42, Cigarettes and Chew.

2. Avoid breathing in irritants.

As much as possible, don't breathe in fumes, toxins, secondhand smoke or dust. Not wearing a respirator doesn't make you tough—it makes you more likely to acquire a chronic lung ailment.

3. Avoid colds, viruses and infections.

For those with COPD, the common cold can lead to serious illness. So wash your hands frequently, especially during cold season. And keep your distance from sick friends.

4. Get vaccinated.

If you have a serious lung disease or are at particular risk for one, get a flu and/ or pneumonia vaccine. You have only two lungs—protect them.

5. Get a "clean" dental checkup before entering the hospital, and brush and floss your teeth immediately before surgery.

Reducing your bacterial load can lower your risk of aspirating bacteria when you are intubated for general anesthesia.

Blabber Mouth!

SECTION 5

THE ORAL ACCESSORY TO MORE DISEASES

IN SECTION 4, YOU LEARNED ABOUT THE LINK between oral health and the Top 5 Killers in America. But that's not where the story ends—because the link between oral and systemic health extends to scores of diseases. Some that you may not suspect include Alzheimer's disease, osteoporosis and Sjögren's syndrome.

We discuss one of the most critical diseases in Chapter 16, Obesity. Although named an official disease only last year, it contributes to every one of the Top 5 Killers. But why is having too much fat on and in our bodies so debilitating? The short answer is simply that fat cells might be big, but they're not lazy. Read on to find out what they do and how you can stop them.

Then we'll switch gears and get back to a topic we discussed in Chapter 10, Traveling Bacteria. If you have any doubt that what begins in the mouth can move to other sites in the body, read the heartbreaking story that starts Chapter 17, Pregnancy Complications. You'll discover that the most common mouth sign of pregnancy, one that impacts up to 75 percent of women, could be the cause of untold numbers of adverse pregnancy outcomes, including preterm and stillbirths.

Traveling bacteria also figure in Chapter 18, Joint Infections. Each year, more than 1 million Americans undergo joint replacement surgeries, most often for new hips and knees. But taking away the synovial fluid that protects the joint, and introducing a foreign body—the artificial joint—creates a risk of infection. And the mouth is a recognized source of bacteria that can cause these infections. So how to prevent them? That's a complex question with an answer that will remain murky until researchers provide more clear and compelling evidence.

Chapter 16

OBESITY: CHEWING THE FAT

NOT LONG AGO, SCIENTISTS BELIEVED fat cells had only one function: to store and release fat. And from the dawn of time, that function has ensured human survival during the cycle of feast and famine.

It's the height of summer when berries, nuts, seeds and wild game are plentiful? Store fat. It's late winter and you're parsing out your last bits of dried salmon and vegetables? Release fat, quickly, before you starve.

Only in recent centuries—and especially in the last 30 years—have societies enjoyed such an abundance of food that the storage of fat began outpacing the release. The result? An upsurge in the number of people who are obese or overweight. The World Health Organization (WHO) estimates that worldwide more than 1 billion adults are overweight and 300 million of those are obese.

What's the objection to being fat? Some may make an aesthetic argument, but not all cultures believe skinny is sexy. Ask the King of Tonga. But the real concern is that obesity doesn't exist in isolation. The risk of other chronic diseases—from type 2 diabetes, heart disease and stroke to cancer, arthritis and periodontitis—surges with increased weight.

The question is *Why*? If fat is just a place to store excess energy, why would it contribute to so many other diseases?

The answer, learned only recently, is that storing energy is only part of fat's job. Fat may be fat, but it doesn't just sit there passively—in fact, it's downright aggressive.

Impact of obesity

In June 2013, the American Medical Association (AMA) officially recognized obesity as a disease. The membership hoped the decision would focus attention on the fight against type 2 diabetes and heart disease, which are both linked to obesity. And as the AMA is fully aware, the problems of obesity are escalating.

According to the Centers for Disease Control and Prevention (CDC), 33.9 percent of Americans are overweight and another 35.1 percent are obese. Add those numbers together and you make the startling conclusion that only 31 percent of us are at a healthy weight.

That made Dr. Susan's words especially poignant when she recently asked, "Have we forgotten what normal is?"

The truth is, there's a new normal, one defined by 155 million Americans who exceed the CDC's guidelines for weight. Those guidelines are admittedly simplistic: Basically they tell us that if your Body Mass Index (BMI) is between 25 and 29.9, you're overweight; above that, you're obese.

You can find BMI calculators on the Web, so we won't get into how to convert your weight into kilograms and square your height in centimeters, which is what the formula demands. You'll also find charts online that will help you determine whether you're underweight, healthy weight, overweight or obese.

It's certainly true that a percentage of the people who exceed the CDC's guidelines on the low end are healthy. The problem is, that's a small percentage—and no matter how much we support embracing your size, whatever it is, as a country we seem to be cuddling up to an unhealthy future.

If obesity rates continue on their current uptick, the number of new cases of type 2 diabetes, coronary heart disease and stroke, high blood pressure and arthritis could increase 10-fold between 2010 and 2020—and double again by 2040. That's according to a 2012 report by the Robert Wood Johnson Foundation.

In fact, the medical costs for patients who are obese run $1,429 per year higher than for those who are healthy weight or even overweight. That increase is about the same amount as the additional cost for smokers.

The impact of obesity on our healthcare system will get worse if the current trends in childhood obesity continue. By 2012, 18 percent of children 6 to 11 years of age were obese, as were 21 percent of adolescents 12 to 19 years of age, according to the National Center for Health Statistics.

This should not be normal.

How obesity happens

Let's talk a little more about the rise and fall of fat in our bodies. The cycle starts when you pull your chair up to the table or your car up to the drive-thru window for a day's worth of calories in a supersized meal. Your body takes in food and breaks it down to send it into the bloodstream. Depending on whether or not you need energy right now, your body either burns your meal for fuel or stores it for the future.

You're taking in fat, carbohydrates and protein, but your body has a different plan for each one. If you're healthy, when you eat your blood sugar rises. In response, your pancreas secretes a hormone called insulin. Hormones are just chemical messengers that tell various parts of the body what to do. Insulin sends a message to cells in your fat tissue, muscles and liver to absorb the energy.

Fat contains 9 calories per gram; protein and carbohydrates, including sugars, each contain 4 calories per gram. So you might think that fat is the biggest culprit when it comes to obesity. But as it turns out, all calories are not created equal. Depending on where they come from, calories have different physiological effects on the body. For the most part, fats break down into triglycerides, protein to amino acids and carbohydrates to glucose, which every cell in your body can use for fuel.

But processed or refined carbs, including sugar, don't work quite so neatly. Table sugar contains equal parts glucose and fructose, and only the liver can break down fructose. The result of the breakdown? Triglyceride. Did you just say, *Wait! Isn't that just like fat?* Thanks for paying attention. You can read more about this process and how it triggered the obesity epidemic in Chapter 43, Sugar.

For now, let's look at what happens when you store fat. You're probably accustomed to thinking of fat as the padding that makes your jeans tight or your shirt buttons gap. That's *subcutaneous* fat—which literally means under the skin. But more dangerous is the visceral fat you can't see, which is stored around internal organs like your heart, liver, kidneys and pancreas.

Fat deposition varies from person to person, but where you store your fat matters. And belly fat means more fat around your vital organs. That's why your waist-to-hip ratio is a measure of risk for life-threatening diseases such as heart disease and stroke, high blood pressure and type 2 diabetes. So pears—those of you with a smaller tummy, bigger butt and legs—have a more healthy shape than apples—bigger tummy, smaller butt and legs.

So how do you lose fat? A good start is to cut sugar and junk-carbohydrate consumption, so you stop storing so much fat. Most experts agree that improving your diet is the key. But another critical element in losing fat is to boost your energy needs—in other words, you need to get moving. When you need energy, hormones send signals to cells in your fat tissue, liver and muscle telling your body to release energy for fuel. That means you lose fat. Generally the number of fat cells stays the same, but the amount of fat stored within each one decreases and the fat cells get smaller.

If you're one of the 69 percent of Americans who are overweight or obese, losing fat is good, as long as you do it slowly. Too much, too soon, and your body will think you're starving—triggering it to do everything it can, including slowing down your metabolism, to start storing fat again.

Oral health and obesity

So far we haven't explained why obesity is associated with so many diseases, from type 2 diabetes to cardiovascular disease to cancer. The reason is that fat doesn't just sit there—it's actually an active substance that secretes hormones called adipokines into the circulatory system. Although fat secretes a number of adipokines, we'll talk about the best-known one only: leptin.

Leptin acts directly on the hypothalamus—a regulator in our brains—to influence food intake. Most obese people have high levels of leptin. So what's the problem? The problem is that with increasing concentrations, leptin prompts cells to become resistant to its actions. Leptin resistance impairs sugar and fat metabolism, resulting in weight gain.

In addition, chronic junk carb and sugar consumption stimulates continual insulin spiking. When the hormone insulin works as it should, it triggers the body's cells to take up sugar from the blood and store it in the liver and muscle as glycogen, which can be used for energy later. While insulin remains high, the body does not use fat as an energy source. So insulin turns off fat burning and turns on fat storage—which can contribute to obesity if it occurs continually.

Insulin spiking may also lead to insulin resistance, in which muscle, fat and liver cells can no longer easily absorb glucose from the bloodstream. The body needs higher and higher levels of insulin, which the pancreas tries to produce. When the pancreas can no longer pump out enough insulin, the excess glucose in the blood can lead to prediabetes, type 2 diabetes and other serious health disorders.

But that's not all. A March 2013 article in *Cell Metabolism* reported on a study by scientists at Houston Methodist Hospital. They found that a high-calorie diet, coupled with excess leptin, causes fat cells to act like they're being attacked. The result? They exhibit an inflammatory response, calling for help. Local immune cells respond to the distress cry, promoting inflammation throughout the body. As you learned in Section 3, inflammation damages arteries and increases susceptibility to a rash of diseases, including periodontitis.

Gum health isn't the only mouth condition at stake, however. Most overweight and obese people don't get that way by overloading on lean protein, fruits, vegetables and whole grains. Instead, a diet full of sweet and starchy snacks and sugary beverages leads to more tooth decay and missing teeth.

Obesity-related diseases often require prescription drugs, many of which cause dry mouth, another factor in increasing tooth decay and periodontal disease. And if you're overweight you're likely to suffer from acid reflux as well, which can erode enamel and promote decay.

According to an article published by the Obesity Action Coalition, studies show that obese individuals have more oral health problems than other individuals. They may have more tooth decay and missing teeth, and fewer dental fillings even though they need them. More of these individuals visit a dentist only when they have a critical issue and not for preventive care.

Evidence of a link

Several studies have shown links between periodontitis and being overweight or obese. As an example, a 2009 study published in *Journal of Clinical Periodontology* showed that overweight adults in Jordan had double the incidence of periodontitis; obese individuals had triple the incidence. Khader and his colleagues looked specifically at BMI, high fat percentage and high waist circumference, and found only the first two significantly associated with an increased risk of periodontitis.

A *Journal of Periodontology* article reported on a study of overweight and obese adults in Brazil. The researchers found obesity significantly associated with periodontitis in non-smoking women. They did not, however, find the same relationship either with women who were overweight but not obese or with men.

A study on the association between obesity and periodontal status among Iranian adults 18 to 34 years of age found that both overall and abdominal obesity were associated with the extent of periodontal disease. The researchers concluded that preventing and managing obesity may be one way to improve periodontal health.

Restoring health

We could talk here about diet and exercise and ways to lose weight and get healthy, but we'll be honest—you've probably heard it all before. We've summed up that information in Quickstart to health.

Here we're going to talk about a new line of defense against obesity, a group of professionals who can help medical doctors fight a disease that the WHO calls an epidemic. They're called dentists and dental hygienists.

When people ask Dr. Susan if she thinks dentists and hygienists should address obesity prevention and intervention in patients, her answer is an unqualified *Yes!* She feels strongly that the dental profession should address this growing epidemic. Given the ongoing preventive relationships most dental teams establish with their patients, they have an excellent opportunity to make a significant difference in patients' overall health, including weight reduction.

But it's a difficult subject to broach. And dentists aren't the only ones who face this issue: Most healthcare providers struggle with how to talk with patients about managing weight through behavior modification. Medical offices have established guidelines that make BMI screening a regular occurrence at every preventive visit, using the results to discuss weight and its impact on overall health, according to the American Heart Association, American College of Cardiology and the Obesity Society.

So how do dentists feel about addressing obesity? It's a hot topic. A recent research article (cover story of the November 2010 *Journal of the American Dental Association*) took stock of dentists' attitudes toward addressing obesity intervention in patients. Their views were divided. Half of dentists (50.3 percent) want to be involved and to develop behaviors, skills and models to make a difference. But currently fewer than 2 percent of general dentists and 5 percent of pediatric dentists offer any diagnosis, discussion or solution-based services around obesity.

In the *JADA* article, the top three fears dentists and hygienists face in talking to patients about obesity are fear of offending patients (54 percent), appearing judgmental (52 percent) and lack of adequate training (46 percent).

There is a growing need for continuing education to help all healthcare professionals be sensitive and non-judgmental when they address obesity. Dentists say they want more competency—access to appropriate models, within the scope of the dental practice, that are clear and effective for patients.

Every significant change begins with a small step. But when it comes to fighting a problem as serious and widespread as obesity, we all need to take responsibility for supporting people with the disease and doing everything we can to promote a healthy lifestyle.

Quickstart to health

1. Calculate your BMI and decide if a change is in order.

Google the term Body Mass Index and use one of the many calculators. Of course, this requires knowing your height and weight—and that requires, gasp, stepping on the scale. Do it!

2. If you're not obese, keep it that way.

Strive to eat a diet that consists of nutrient-rich whole foods and to exercise at least five days each week for at least 30 minutes.

3. If you're overweight, change your diet.

You knew we'd say that. Where to begin? Start by cutting out sweetened or diet beverages. Cut all processed, sugar-added, salty, crunchy snacks—the ones with lots of empty calories—because they lead to binging. (You may think the co-authors of this book are immune to cravings, but they're not. Diana will eat every single last chip, no matter how small or big the bag.) Increase your fiber by replacing junk carbs with vegetables, fruits, nuts and seeds. You'll lose fat and increase vitamins, minerals and micronutrients.

4. Get moving.

You know this too. To increase your calorie expenditure, take a walk or run. Use the stairs if you're headed to the 3rd floor or below. Also increase weight-bearing activity to build muscle, because muscle burns more than three times the calories that fat does, even when it's just resting. Find an activity you like—yoga, ice skating, jazz dance—and lose a little fat while you give your lungs and heart something to be happy about.

5. Talk with your healthcare professional.

Face it: It's hard for physicians and dentists to bring up the subject of your weight. They may worry about offending you. Ask for their help in achieving a healthy weight. Even losing a small percentage of excess weight can greatly reduce your risk of many chronic diseases, including periodontal disease.

6. Be smart about choosing community and commercial weight management programs.

Many people find it easier to lose weight in a community with others who face the same issue, and provide accountability and emotional support. But make sure the program promotes healthful eating for a lifetime, not just a quick weight-loss fix.

Chapter 17

PREGNANCY COMPLICATIONS: A STARTLING CAUSE

JUST DAYS SHORT OF HER DUE DATE, a 35-year-old Asian woman was admitted to Saint John's Health Center in Santa Monica, California. For three days, she'd been mildly ill with a respiratory tract infection and low-grade fever. But her pregnancy had been uncomplicated up to that point: no fluid leakage, no bleeding, no abnormal contractions. She did, however, have excessive gum bleeding from the most common mouth sign of pregnancy—gingivitis.

The morning she entered the hospital, the mother felt her baby move at about 5 a.m. After that, nothing. Once admitted, ultrasound confirmed the lack of a fetal heartbeat. Her doctor ruptured the amniotic sac and delivered a stillborn female.

The baby had died due to a massive infection. Doctors often think that infections in the fetal-placental unit are triggered by bacteria transmitted from the vaginal or colorectal tract. But the bacteria found, *Fusobacterium nucleatum*, was not present in either of those areas. Instead, studies conducted by dental bacteria researcher Dr. Yiping Han and her colleagues determined that the bacteria initiated in the mother's mouth. The bacteria may have moved to the uterus while the mom's immune system was weakened during her respiratory infection. Dr. Han's study provided the first evidence in humans that oral bacteria could result in a uterine infection that moved to the placenta, the amniotic fluid and to the unborn baby, causing death.

One other note: Although evidence shows a link between periodontitis and pregnancy complications, a dental exam three weeks later showed that this mother did not have periodontitis—only pregnancy gingivitis. If you pick up a what-to-expect book on pregnancy, you'll see that it's reported among at least 75 percent of pregnant women. But what was not known until recently is that you could deliver prematurely, have a low birthweight baby or even lose your child due to this common gum infection.

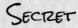

The impact of pregnancy complications

Oral health has been associated with various types of pregnancy complications, from stillbirth, preterm birth and low birthweight to miscarriage and preeclampsia (high blood pressure and fluid retention in the mother). These complications may cause the baby's death, either before birth or within the first year of life. Even if the baby lives, over his lifetime he may deal with respiratory issues, impaired motor skills, delayed development, and visual and learning difficulties. We'll focus here on three complications: stillbirth, preterm birth and low birthweight.

Stillbirth is fetal death before 20 weeks of pregnancy and occurs in one in 160 pregnancies. In the United States, 26,000 babies are stillborn each year; worldwide the number is 2.6 million.

Preterm birth is the live birth of an infant before the 37th week of pregnancy. Around the world, more than 15 million babies—one in 10 live births—are born too soon every year. More than 1 million children die each year due to complications from this early birth.

Low birthweight, which occurs in one in 10 babies, is often the result of being born before full term. But babies may also not gain the weight they should before birth. These babies weigh less than 5 pounds and 8 ounces, one-third less than the average 7-pound infant. This low weight is a predictor for future disease and death—and the lower the weight, the more challenges occur.

How still and preterm birth and low birthweight happen

Stillbirth can result from birth defects, placental problems, poor fetal growth, chronic health conditions and umbilical cord accidents. But also significant are infections—involving either the mother, fetus or placenta—that cause 10 percent to 25 percent of stillbirths.

Preterm birth occurs for three primary reasons. In about 20 percent of cases, a physician decides to deliver the baby early due to problems experienced by the mother or child, such as high blood pressure or fetal distress. In the rest, preterm births result either from spontaneous onset of labor or premature rupture of the membranes.

The two primary causes of low birthweight babies are high blood pressure and diabetes. But heart, lung and kidney problems are also major issues.

The role of oral health

To understand the role of oral health in pregnancy complications, it's important to know that inflammatory signals control normal pregnancies and deliveries. When it's time for a baby to be born, signals from inflammatory markers reach a critical point and trigger water breaking, contractions, cervical dilation and delivery. But all this can happen prematurely if the mom has infection and inflammation. An increased level of C-reactive protein, a marker of systemic inflammation that's appeared throughout **BlabberMouth!**, has been associated with an increased risk for pregnancy complications.

We've discussed periodontitis as a source of inflammation and oral bacteria in Chapters 9 and 10. But it's now clear that pregnancy gingivitis may also be a source. During pregnancy, levels of the hormone progesterone increase, making it easier for gingivitis-causing bacteria to grow and cause an infection. Pregnancy hormones also create a hyper-response to the inflammatory toxins that result from the mom's oral plaque. Not surprisingly then, the two main mechanisms that link gum disease with pregnancy complications are inflammation and traveling bacteria from an infection.

In the first mechanism, which is an indirect pathway, inflammatory markers that are produced as a response to a gum infection can enter the bloodstream. These markers may reach the liver and stimulate a system-wide inflammatory response. Or they might move to the placenta, where they could trigger the production of prostaglandin and signal the start of labor.

In the second mechanism, a direct pathway, oral bacteria travel via the bloodstream and cause an infection in the uterus, which moves to the placenta, amniotic sac and ultimately the baby. The bacteria may colonize these distant locations, resulting in infection, inflammation and devastating outcomes. Studies in animal models have shown that oral bacteria can cause both chronic and acute infections in the placenta.

Evidence of a link

In 2013, Ide and Papapanou conducted the most recent systematic review of the association between oral health and pregnancy complications. They concluded that a positive association exists between poor maternal periodontal status and three adverse pregnancy outcomes: preterm birth, low birthweight and preeclampsia.

In addition, this chapter began with evidence linking stillbirth to the periodontal bacteria *F. nucleatum,* circulating in the blood, leading to infection and inflammation of the membranes, placenta and fetus. This discovery makes the case for a scientific re-evaluation of conventional thinking on infections of the uterus. Current thought is that the source of these infections is vaginal bacteria that creeps up and into the otherwise sterile uterus. But now that researchers can identify specific bacteria using advanced DNA techniques, other sources of bacteria, including the mouth, are coming to light.

Evidence is growing that oral bacteria may move directly into the pregnant uterus, causing localized inflammation there, which negatively affects the pregnancy. Future studies will investigate the mechanisms of that infection and also the mother's susceptibility to this oral-uterine transmission. Scientists need to better understand these mechanisms to establish meaningful strategies to prevent transmission.

So what can be done now to prevent these complications? The answer to that question is not clear. Studies have shown that nonsurgical treatment of gum disease during the second trimester does not result in a decreased rate of preterm delivery or have a positive impact on birthweight.

For now, just like every other part of the body, a woman should have her mouth in optimal health before she conceives—and then practice meticulous oral hygiene throughout her pregnancy.

Quickstart to health

1. See the dentist at least twice a year.

We all need a complete periodontal evaluation every year and treatment for gum disease, if we have it. But if you're a woman planning to conceive, take particular care to make sure your mouth is as healthy as possible before you get pregnant. If you've had gum disease, you should have a periodontal maintenance visit every three months.

2. Practice meticulous oral hygiene.

This is good advice for all of us. But women who are planning to get pregnant or who already are should make even greater efforts to keep their mouths clean by brushing and flossing at least twice a day.

Chapter 18

JOINT INFECTIONS: NEW TERRITORY FOR BACTERIA

From the chair

CHAR SAW ME FOR A NEW-PATIENT EMERGENCY—*a raging toothache. She was not only in pain but concerned that any dental procedure might delay the shoulder replacement surgery she had scheduled for the following week. After examining her and taking x-rays, I identified an infected, abscessed tooth, as well as chronic active gum disease. I then helped Char and her orthopedic surgeon understand the importance of postponing the elective prosthetic joint surgery until her mouth infections were stabilized.*

The impact of joint infections

Joint replacements are among the most common elective surgeries today. They can seem like a miracle cure for an often sedentary and pain-filled life. Every year, U.S. surgeons replace more than 1 million knees, hips, shoulders, elbows and ankles. Of those, knees and hips are the most common. A 2014 Mayo Clinic study reported some 4.7 million artificial knees and 2.5 million artificial hips among U.S. adults.

As an aside, the Mayo researchers presented their findings at the American Academy of Orthopaedic Surgeons (AAOS) 2014 meeting and forecasted the need for the healthcare system to prepare for special continued care of an aging population with an ever-increasing number of prosthetic joints.

Although commonplace, no surgery goes without risk, especially one that places a foreign object into the body and intends it for long-term integration. So you may not be surprised that in one in 100 joint replacement surgeries, the patient will develop a bacterial infection at some point after the surgery. Some infections occur as soon as a few days post-surgery and some develop years later.

Treating these infections, which requires another surgery and targeted antibiotic therapy, may result in significantly greater disability than the original failing joint. Complications include blood infection and even death.

Although the risk is considered small, research shows that as many as 23 percent of joint replacement patients have dental infection that could result in joint infection. Let's take a look at how that occurs.

How joint infections happen

For bacteria to grow at the site of a replacement joint, it must enter the body, travel within it and end up on the joint itself. Threatening bacteria most commonly enter the body through breaks or cuts in the skin, in urinary or respiratory tract infections, through wounds from other surgeries or, of course, from infections in the mouth.

With intruding bacteria in the body, your 24/7 immune system recruits a patrol of white blood cells to destroy and clean up the intruders. But if the dangerous bugs become too heavy a load to handle, some of the bacteria may escape and travel within your body. (See Chapter 10, Traveling Bacteria, for a full discussion.)

Other factors may come into play as well to prevent a full bacterial clean-up. For example, if you have human immunodeficiency virus, cancer, diabetes, obesity or poor peripheral blood circulation, your immune system is already taxed and might not get the job done.

But why would a prosthetic joint serve as a home for oral and other bacteria?

"The reasons why are many and complex, but first, joint replacement, by default, removes most of the joint lining (synovium), which ordinarily serves as a natural barrier to infection," says Dr. Christoper Bibbo, Chief, Foot & Ankle, Limb Preservation & Microsurgery Department of Orthopedics, Marshfield Clinic, Marshfield, Wisconsin. "Second, even the most advanced joint implant is still recognized as a foreign body; it has microscopic surface roughness (for bone attachment) to which bacteria might adhere and multiply."

The reason Dr. Susan urged Char to postpone her shoulder replacement is that these secondary infections most commonly result from active periodontal disease, but may also occur from unresolved pulp-death infections (an abscess) or even the more superficial gum infection, acute gingivitis. Char had all three.

The role of oral health

Many studies have confirmed that infections in artificial joints have been seeded by dangerous strains of oral bacteria associated with gum disease and pulp abscesses. But what if you don't have either of those but need an invasive dental procedure, like an extraction or root canal? Or even a noninvasive procedure, like a cleaning?

The view on how to manage dental procedures to protect patients who have had joint replacements changed recently. For decades all dental patients with joint replacements were routinely prescribed antibiotic coverage before all dental appointments, even professional cleanings. That's because dental instruments may cause micro-breaks in the gum tissue, opening a portal through which oral bacteria could travel. And invasive procedures make it that much easier for bacteria to reach the bloodstream.

From there the risk of prosthetic joint infection varies depending on a range of factors, including the individual patient's age, other diseases such as diabetes, nutritional deficits and the ability to fight infection.

But the 2013 recommendations by the American Dental Association (ADA) and AAOS changed the practice of pre-medicating patients with antibiotics. We'll explain that in much more detail in the next section. What hasn't changed is the collective understanding that dentists need to stop any and all oral infection before patients undergo an elective joint replacement surgery.

SECRET

Addressing oral infection and establishing a healthy mouth before joint replacement surgery may make the difference between normal healing and secondary infection from oral bacteria.

Evidence of a link

Based on the evidence available at the time, in 2009 the AAOS released a new statement on pre-medicating patients with joint replacements: "Given the potential adverse outcomes and cost of treating an infected joint replacement, the AAOS recommends that clinicians consider antibiotic prophylaxis (pre-medication) for all total joint replacement patients prior to any invasive dental procedure that may cause bacteremia."

But every few years, the AAOS reevaluates the dental guidelines. As evidence changes, the AAOS must weigh the most current studies that link oral bacteria to prosthetic joint infections against the ever-growing health threat of antibiotic coverage.

Widespread use of antibiotics brings the health risk of adverse or allergic reactions, increased cost and, more importantly, the increased risk that the bacteria are resistant to antibiotics. In today's world, antibiotic-resistant bugs, also called "superbugs," continue to cast a dark shadow on the miracle cures that antibiotics have historically offered. Medical science is slowly responding.

In 2012, the AAOS along with the ADA abolished the standing guidelines that called for antibiotic coverage for any dental procedure carried out within two years of joint replacement surgery. They noted that those guidelines were based on a single 1986 study that showed the greatest risk for prosthetic joint infection was for two years following surgery—but that alone wasn't enough evidence.

Still it surprised the medical and dental community when the 2012 AAOS-ADA guidelines stated that there is not enough reasonable data to support the belief that the bacteria entering the bloodstream following dental procedures had a direct link to the risk of prosthetic joint infections. Now the risks of antibiotic coverage seemed to outweigh the benefits for preventing infections.

The guidelines were widely criticized as being too ambiguous, leaving the antibiotic recommendation largely in the hands of the dentist and/or orthopedic surgeon without clear direction. So in 2013, the ADA Council on Scientific Affairs formed a panel to study three more substantial studies. They reached a conclusion based on the risk to the patient.

> ## SECRET
>
> **Antibiotic protection during a dental visit is no longer necessary for most patients with a prosthetic joint, unless they have some other serious health consideration that threatens their immunity (such as diabetes, rheumatoid arthritis, cancer, chemotherapy, or chronic steroid use).**

If you do have health considerations that impact your immune response, then preventive antibiotics are considered critical to protect you from prosthetic joint infections seeded by oral bacteria. That calls for your orthopedic surgeon and dentist to collaborate and periodically re-establish your protection plan.

Dr. Susan reports from her clinical experience that many orthopedic surgeons, when consulted, still opt for a lifetime of antibiotic prophylaxis to avoid the threat of oral bacterial infection. The ADA recommends that dentists make thoughtful judgments based on the individual patient and current guidelines, and not opt out of the decision on antibiotics by passing it to the orthopedic surgeon. The dentist better understands the invasiveness of scheduled procedures and should also be aware of the patient's current health challenges.

With guidelines changing so frequently, in response to the growing body of evidence around prosthetic joint infection as well as antibiotic over-use, the next few years are likely to bring further changes in best practices.

Quickstart to health

1. If you're planning any joint surgery, make sure you're in optimal oral health first.

Get a thorough oral health examination and treat any existing infection that might pose a threat to the success of your surgery.

2. If you have a prosthetic joint but no specific health threats, skip routine antibiotic coverage.

Reserving antibiotics for when they are medically necessary will reduce your risk of adverse reaction and your chance of antibiotic resistance.

3. If you have a prosthetic joint and special health threats, consult your doctors for a protection plan.

Talk to both your dentist and your orthopedic surgeon to establish a protection plan. You always benefit from collaboration between your health professionals, because the guidelines change frequently, as does your health. Urge your docs to review your protection plan at least every two years.

SECTION 6
OTHER DISEASE LINKS

EVER PLAY DOCTOR AS A KID? Really, we don't want to know. But we do want to give you a chance to play dentist now that you're an adult. So let's give your diagnostic skills a try.

What disease or condition would you suspect if you noted the following in a patient?

- A deep overbite, a turkey waddle and a narrow opening to the back of the throat?

- A sticky mouth and bad breath?

- Enamel eroding off the tops and tongue side of the teeth?

Any guesses? As it turns out, not all ailments associated with oral health include a role for inflammation and infection. Some result from other causes—and frequently it's your dentist who diagnoses them first from telltale signs on your gums, teeth, tongue and throat.

In this section, we'll discuss three diseases you can learn about just by looking in the mouth—and, in no particular order, they're the answers to our diagnostic quiz above:

- Obstructive Sleep Apnea, which contributes to other serious diseases and can lead to sudden death, as we'll discuss in Chapter 19;

- Acid Reflux, which can be a precursor to cancer if left untreated, as we explain in Chapter 20;

- Cotton Mouth, a common condition underlying rampant tooth decay and gum disease, as you'll learn in Chapter 21.

Chapter 19

Obstructive Sleep Apnea: From Snoring to Cardio Disease

WE ALL KNOW THAT SNORING CAN BE A NUISANCE; in fact, we talk about snoring and its potential to derail your sex life in Chapter 32, Snoring. But worse still, snoring can be a red flag of Obstructive Sleep Apnea (OSA), which can shorten your life by many years.

How OSA happens

During the day, you don't usually have to think about keeping your airway open as you go about your business. But at night, as you slip into restful Rapid Eye Movement (REM) sleep, a growing number of dozers can't keep their airways open. During REM sleep your eyes move, but the rest of your skeletal muscles are paralyzed.

That's normal. But if throat tissues block your airway, you stop breathing. That's called *apnea*, from Greek words that mean no breathing. That's not so normal. Soon the brain picks up the emergency "Poison!!!" alert from the buildup of carbon dioxide (CO_2) and wakes you up in time to offload CO_2 and suck in a fresh breath of air.

Then the cycle repeats, anywhere from a few times an hour to more than once a minute. Of course, the oxygen deprivation during these apnea events is dangerous to the brain and your other organs too.

Warning signs of OSA

The American Sleep Apnea Association (ASAA) estimates that 22 million Americans (4 percent of men and 2 percent of women) suffer from sleep apnea. Both snoring and OSA are on the rise, mostly thanks to the ever-increasing obesity rate.

If you have OSA, you generally don't know you're waking up constantly during the night. But even if you're in bed for the recommended seven or eight hours, you'll be getting a lot less sleep. Symptoms of sleep deprivation include fatigue, irritability, depression, reduced attention, concentration and memory, frequent illnesses, lost productivity, and workplace or auto accidents. In fact, the National Highway Traffic Safety Administration estimates that more than 100,000 accidents each year may be related to sleepiness.

If you lose just 90 minutes of REM sleep a night, your cognitive ability drops off 35 percent the next day. To maintain your memory, processing speed and problem-solving ability, have a sleep test if you suspect you have OSA.

Other symptoms related to sleep deprivation can be even more damaging to your health. When left untreated, sleep apnea can lead to high blood pressure, chronic heart failure, atrial fibrillation, stroke and other cardiovascular problems. OSA is also associated with type 2 diabetes and depression.

Although you can have OSA without being overweight and be overweight without having OSA, you can't ignore that obesity—especially abdominal fat—is a big risk factor for OSA. Individuals who don't sleep well find it harder to lose weight. Scientists once thought that OSA sufferers eat more because their energy is low, but more recent studies reported in the *European Respiratory Journal* show that OSA negatively influences the hunger hormones leptin and ghrelin.

Secret

Overweight or obese individuals with OSA face a vicious cycle. Excess weight makes OSA more likely; and OSA makes it harder to lose weight. The best option to improve your health is to tackle both at the same time.

Your risk of OSA

To determine if you're at risk for OSA, you can start with an assessment using Dr. Susan's self-screening tool. To take the test electronically or to share it with others, just go to http://SelfScreen.net or use the QR code below.

OSA Risk Assessment

Scoring: Yes=2 points, Occasionally=1 point, No=0 points

_____ Do you smoke?

_____ Do you drink alcohol close to bedtime?

_____ Have you been told you snore?

_____ When you get seven to eight hours of sleep, are you still fatigued or sleepy during the day?

_____ Do you have morning headaches?

_____ Are you more than 10 percent above ideal body weight?

_____ Do you have difficulty losing weight?

_____ Do you have high blood pressure?

_____ Do you have acid reflux?

_____ Do you have insomnia?

_____ Do you take any antidepressants or sleep aids?

_____ Do you have difficulty remembering names?

_____ Do you experience or take medications for erectile dysfunction?

_____ **Total points**

Score total points:

1-3 Very low risk of OSA: Learn more about prevention

4-6 Low risk of OSA: Make lifestyle changes

7-10 Moderate risk of OSA: Consult your physician

11+ High risk of OSA: See your physician immediately

If your risk of OSA is moderate to high, we suggest you ask your physician for a referral to a sleep-medicine practice for an accurate diagnosis.

Restoring health

A major issue in treating OSA is that it's rarely recognized as a problem: Some 80 percent of moderate and severe cases of OSA go undiagnosed, according to ASAA. In fact, most physicians who are not sleep specialists do not even screen for OSA.

Dentists are in an ideal position to screen for OSA, because they can identify physical risk factors besides obesity. The signs that a dental patient has OSA include a deep overbite (upper teeth that hide the lower teeth when biting down), a small "cricomental space" in the neck (otherwise known as a turkey waddle) and a narrowed airway opening to the back of the throat. If you have all three of these physical factors, your risk of sleep apnea is 85 percent.

Your dentist will assess the size of your throat opening based on the *Mallampati* classification. If you'd like to make an assessment yourself, look in the mirror and open your mouth normally, without saying *Ahhhhhh*. Then compare your throat opening with the illustrations below. Class III and IV are associated with a higher incidence of OSA.

Measuring cricomental space

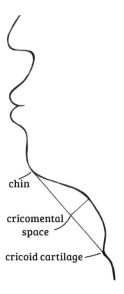

chin

cricomental space

cricoid cartilage

Mallampati classification

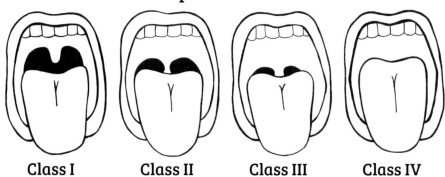

| Class I | Class II | Class III | Class IV |

Diagnosing OSA accurately requires a "sleep study." For this study, sleep technicians fit you with simple equipment to check a variety of factors, including blood oxygen levels, respiration rate, brain-wave activity, leg movements and the apnea-hypopnea index. This index is a measure of sleep apnea severity based on the number of times you don't breathe (apnea) or breathe shallowly (hypopnea) within each hour. Sleep studies are often done in a sleep lab, which is a glorified hotel room, but they can also be done in your home, if you're more comfortable with that.

Dr. Susan has noticed that even if a patient suspects OSA in himself or his partner, he may not want a sleep study for diagnosis. Why not? Because he may have heard about or seen Continuous Positive Airway Pressure (CPAP) machines commonly used to treat OSA and doesn't want anything to do with them. These combination box-hose-mask devices blow a constant stream of air into your nose, which keeps your airway open.

But less intrusive alternatives exist. If you're diagnosed with mild or moderate OSA, an oral appliance can help open your airway at night. Oral appliances consist of two pieces that work together. One fits precisely on the upper teeth, the other on the lower. Together they hold the lower jaw forward. This opens the airway in a position you might be familiar with if you've had training in mouth-to-mouth resuscitation.

Surgery to create a larger airway by repositioning the jaw and/or removing tissue is also an option. This can be done by widening the upper arch of the jaw or moving it forward, moving the lower jaw forward or removing some soft tissue from the back of the soft palate. Many people view surgery as a radical measure—but the choice may be a lifetime of using a CPAP machine or of living with a serious threat to your overall health.

A new FDA-approved treatment for OSA may be promising if you can't tolerate a CPAP machine and don't want an oral appliance or surgery. Upper airway simulation (UAS) therapy uses a small electrode implanted in your body to stimulate the hypoglossal nerve, which moves the tongue. This excites the muscles that support the airway to keep them working even when you sleep.

Quickstart to health

1. Read the first five items in Chapter 32, Snoring, Quickstart to health.

See if the measures listed help alleviate your symptoms. You deserve to sleep well at night and wake up refreshed and ready to take on the day.

2. Agree to a sleep study.

A sleep study can help you get an accurate diagnosis for sleep apnea, so you know if you have the disease and, if so, how much it's interfering with your life.

3. Lose weight.

OSA makes it much more difficult to lose weight. You'll be more successful if you treat the OSA while engaging in a diet and exercise plan rather than trying to lose weight while living with the health threat of OSA. Many of Dr. Susan's patients are shocked at how much easier it is to lose unwanted pounds once OSA is treated.

4. Use a Continuous Positive Airway Pressure (CPAP) device.

Treatments for OSA vary, but one of the most common and effective is the CPAP device. By blowing a constant stream of air into your nose, the CPAP device keeps your airway open and stops the apnea and constant awakenings.

5. Consider an oral appliance.

For patients with mild or moderate OSA who won't tolerate CPAP, the American Academy for Sleep Medicine recommends an oral appliance to help hold the airway open during sleep. As noted in Chapter 32, Snoring, these appliances can be a tolerable and effective solution to snoring and OSA.

6. Consider jaw surgery.

In some cases, creating a larger airway is an effective treatment choice. Although surgery seems like a drastic treatment option, compare that to a lifetime of using a CPAP machine or, even worse, living with the severe threat to your health if you don't treat OSA.

7. Ask about Upper Airway Simulation (UAS) therapy.

This electrode uses a nerve under the tongue to keep the muscles that support the airway awake even when you're asleep.

Chapter 20

Acid Reflux: From Enamel Erosion to Esophageal Cancer

QUESTION: WHICH POP ARTIST blamed a lip-syncing miscue during a "Saturday Night Live" performance on acid reflux?

Multiple choice:

A. Janet Jackson

B. Ashlee Simpson

C. Beyoncé

D. Avril Lavigne

If you got the right answer—B, Ashlee Simpson—then you, like one of the authors of this book, pay far too much attention to pop culture. But the ill effects of acid reflux go far beyond the hoarseness that prompted Simpson to nix a live performance.

Acid reflux affects as many as 40 percent of Americans, according to Dr. Jamie Koufman, a leader in acid reflux treatment and author of *Dropping Acid: The Reflux Diet Cookbook and Cure.* You might know you suffer from acid reflux if you have heartburn or sometimes throw up a little in your mouth. But you may miss it if you have "silent" symptoms, like waking up with a sexier (hoarse) voice than normal, coughing or clearing your throat a lot, or difficulty swallowing.

Dr. Koufman reminds us that reflux has grown at 4 percent a year since 1976, from 10 percent of our adult population to a whopping 40 percent. Why the increase? She believes the main culprits are our unhealthy lifestyles and diets. As a result, sales of prescribed and over-the-counter anti-reflux medications now exceed $13 billion per year.

How acid reflux happens

Acid reflux occurs when pepsin, the stomach acid that helps digest your food, urps up from the stomach. Along the way, it hits the tissue of the esophagus (the 8-inch tube that connects the stomach to the throat), the throat and tonsils, sinuses, lungs and the mouth. You don't have to experience the bitter taste of regurgitation to have pepsin at work eroding your tissue and teeth. Pepsin is a destroyer that causes damage everywhere other than where it's supposed to be—in the stomach.

Most of us don't think about reflux until we have that burning sensation in the chest we call heartburn, which thankfully does not involve the heart. This chest pain comes right from the esophagus and is historically labeled gastroesophageal reflux disease or GERD.

In a recent interview with Dr. Susan, Dr. Koufman said, "The root cause of all this [reflux] is unhealthy eating. The dietary trends in the U.S. include increased saturated fat, increased high-fructose corn syrup, increased exposure to food pollutants and increased dietary acid."

The acid added to our food and drinks has become a major issue. Manufacturers use acid as a food additive to ensure a longer shelflife. But worse still are the beverages we consume, many of which contain startling amounts of acid. In 2010, for example, the average 12- to 29-year-old male consumed 160 gallons of soft drinks each year—about two quarts a day of a liquid that's almost as acidic as stomach acid. How acidic is soda compared to water and saliva, which are neutral? Remember that pH, a measure of acidity, uses a logarithmic scale—so with a pH of 2.9, soda is about 10,000 times as acidic as water and saliva, with a pH of 7.0.

Warning signs of acid reflux

Dr. Koufman said she surveyed a series of 500 reflux patients in her office, and only 17 percent had heartburn as their main complaint. More than half had *never* experienced heartburn. Instead they had the *silent* symptoms we discussed above that, if not recognized, could advance to heartburn or even to cellular changes that result in cancer of the esophagus, throat and tongue.

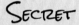

SECRET

By the time you have heartburn, acid reflux is advanced, because it takes a lot of pepsin exposure to damage the esophagus and cause it to "burn." Pay attention to silent symptoms that can warn you of cellular changes that may lead to cancer.

Dr. Susan often sees the telltale signs of reflux in the mouth: disappearing enamel on the tops and tongue side of a patient's teeth. It's even more pronounced if you grind your teeth and you have reflux. This acid comes from a different source than the acid-producing bacteria that cause tooth decay. Still, acid is acid, so pepsin from reflux definitely promotes the decay process. Your saliva, which always works to neutralize the acid, just can't keep up. If you happen to grind your teeth as well, bathing them in acid makes the wear on biting surfaces much worse.

Other symptoms that lead to a diagnosis of reflux—but not acid reflux—include a chronic cough, post-nasal drip, a gravely voice, recurring sinusitis, bronchitis or even asthma. You may have these symptoms but not know what's causing them. They fall under a diagnosis now known as *airway reflux*—stomach acid wreaking havoc with your breathing tubes. Dr. Koufman believes that 80 percent of people diagnosed with asthma in the United States may have been misdiagnosed—and they may have airway reflux instead.

Pathway to cancer

If left untreated, reflux can cause far more serious complications. A 2006 Mayo Clinic study found that 5 percent of people with acid reflux develop Barrett's esophagus, a change in the lining of the tube that is a precursor to cancer. Even before that, the *New England Journal of Medicine* reported in 1999 that patients with chronic, untreated heartburn had a substantially greater risk of developing cancer of the esophagus. Esophageal cancer has increased by about 500 percent since the 1970s, Dr. Koufman reports.

Although this cancer is not common, it is particularly deadly. The National Cancer Institute estimated 16,980 new cases of esophageal cancer in the United States in 2015 and 15,590 deaths from the disease.

That number is growing, in part because acid reflux has almost doubled in the past decade. Researchers in Norway found the number of people reporting symptoms of reflux at least once a week increased 30 percent over a 14-year study, from 31 percent at the beginning to 40 percent at the end.

Why the jump? Obesity and acidification of our food supply. Studies show that people who are obese are more likely to suffer from reflux. The exact mechanism is not known, but it's thought that excess weight may put added pressure on the stomach, forcing acid into the esophagus.

An analysis of the Nurses' Health Study of 10,000 women found that a relatively modest weight gain of 10 to 20 pounds increased the likelihood of heartburn symptoms threefold.

Your risk of acid reflux

To determine if you're at risk for acid reflux, you can start with an assessment using Dr. Susan's self-screening tool. To take the test electronically or to share it with others, just go to http://SelfScreen.net or use the QR code below.

Acid Reflux Risk Assessment

Scoring: Yes=2 points, Occasionally=1 point, No=0 points

_____ Do you smoke?

_____ Are you more than 10 percent above your ideal body weight??

_____ Do you experience frequent heartburn or chest pains (primarily after eating)?

_____ Do you have difficulty breathing or swallowing?

_____ Do you feel as if there is a constant lump in your throat?

_____ Do you experience regurgitation?

_____ Do you experience post-nasal drip or excess throat mucus?

_____ Do you suffer from a chronic cough?

_____ Do you experience frequent choking episodes?

_____ Do you suffer from indigestion, burping, nausea after eating or stomach bloating?

_____ Do you feel hoarseness in your throat, primarily in the mornings?

_____ Are you prone to tooth decay or acid erosion of your enamel?

_____ **Total points**

Score total points:

1-3 Very low risk of reflux or GERD: Learn more about prevention

4-6 Low risk of reflux or GERD: Make lifestyle changes

7-10 Moderate risk of reflux or GERD: Consult your physician

11+ High risk of reflux or GERD: See your physician immediately

If you suspect reflux, treatment options should begin with changes to your lifestyle and diet. Working together, your physician along with your dentist can help you manage acid reflux and protect your teeth.

Restoring health

Anti-reflux medication alone does not appear to control reflux disease. A Danish study published in 2014 concluded that there are no cancer-protective effects from using the common anti-reflux medications, called proton pump inhibitors (PPIs). Regular long-term use was actually associated with an increased risk of developing esophageal cancer.

Avoiding acidic foods and drinks is an obvious step for alleviating reflux. If you're serious about addressing reflux without medication, consider eliminating processed—and by that we mean acid-laden—food entirely. Dr. Susan strongly recommends Dr. Koufman's book *Dropping Acid* to learn more about what and how to eat to alleviate reflux.

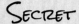

Secret

Losing weight is another change you can make to help reduce reflux without the need for constant medication. Obese people are nearly three times more likely to experience acid reflux as people of normal weight.

Dr. Koufman believes the single most important change is to eliminate late eating, particularly when the meal consists of large portions of over-processed, fatty food. That's often the case because many Americans skip breakfast and eat only a sandwich at lunch. Although Europeans often eat late, their portions generally are much smaller and they experience far less reflux disease.

After eating, staying upright for several hours keeps the content of the meal in the stomach. Lying down on the couch to watch TV, especially on a full stomach, makes reflux much more likely. You can even raise the head of your bed to alleviate acid reflux.

Quickstart to health

1. Change your diet.

First and foremost, avoid soda entirely, sugared or diet. Many soft drinks are as acidic as pepsin. Avoid overeating, especially foods high in acid or hydrogenated (solid) fat or acid, including chocolate, citrus juice and tomato juice.

2. Don't eat within three hours of bedtime.

Much of the damage caused by acid reflux occurs at night, because a horizontal position makes it easier for acid to flow backward. Not eating before bedtime limits the amount of stomach acid available.

3. Lose weight.

Acid reflux is strongly associated with weight gain, so losing weight can alleviate symptoms and improve your overall health.

4. Limit alcohol and avoid smoking.

Not only is alcohol acidic, but both drinking and smoking relax the valve separating the esophagus and stomach, contributing to acid reflux.

5. See your physician for medications.

If changing your diet and lifestyle don't alleviate symptoms, see your physician, who may recommend over-the-counter or prescription medications. Medications for acid reflux include antacids, like Mylanta® or Maalox®, histamine 2-receptor agonists, like Zantac®, and proton pump inhibitors, like Prilosec OTC® or Prevacid®24HR. Your physician can prescribe stronger versions of these medications, if necessary.

6. Consider surgery.

If the natural acid barrier between your stomach and esophagus is compromised, your physician may suggest surgery to repair it.

Chapter 21

Cotton Mouth: From Desert to Disease

Saliva is one of those substances that you may not think much about—unless it's not there. Then you're suddenly only too aware of all the things it does: bathes and lubricates the mouth, helps digest foods, prevents tooth decay and aids in speech and swallowing.

When saliva flows slow down, the result is dry mouth, also called *xerostomia*. Despite the fancy name, this isn't a specific disorder, but rather a side effect of various physical stressors.

Saliva helps prevent tooth decay and gum disease by neutralizing acids produced by bacteria, limiting bacterial growth and washing away food particles. A lack of saliva can send tooth decay and gum disease on a rampage, leading to both emotional and financial distress.

Saliva also boosts your ability to taste food and drink, and makes it easier to swallow. And enzymes in saliva aid in digestion. So it's not surprising that a lack of saliva can impact your appetite and enjoyment of food—and more critically, limit your ability to get adequate nutrition.

> ## Secret
> Saliva neutralizes acids and adds back minerals to teeth weakened by acidic food and drink. But age and unhealthy lifestyles may make saliva more acidic due to deficiency of minerals, especially calcium. Strongly deficient saliva may be a sign of serious disease, including arthritis, osteoporosis and cancer.

How cotton mouth happens

Most often, dry mouth is a side effect of medication you're taking. More than 400 medications list dry mouth as a side effect. These include diuretics, blood pressure meds, antidepressants, pain meds (especially narcotics), antihistamines and decongestants. If you suspect your medications are the root cause of your xerostomia, read the package insert. Then bring it to the attention of your prescribing physician or dentist. Often there are suitable substitutes that will help you regain healthy mouth lubrication.

Dry mouth has many other potential causes too, including autoimmune disorders or disturbances such as Sjögren's syndrome, HIV or diabetes. Other possibilities include radiation treatment for cancer of the head or neck, which destroys salivary gland tissue, at least temporarily. Surgery or trauma to the head and neck can also impact your salivary glands, as can changes in hormone levels like those that occur during menopause.

Warning signs of cotton mouth

When saliva flow slows down, you'll notice a sticky mouth and bad breath. But that's just the beginning. Depending on how dry your mouth is, it can range from being merely a nuisance to creating a major impact on your overall health and the health of your teeth.

More critical signs include tooth decay and gum disease that persist despite diligent home care of your mouth. And you may also notice you struggle to taste your meals, making it more challenging to appreciate one of the great pleasures of life—food and drink.

Restoring health

When your mouth is dry, the first inclination is to suck on candy or chew gum to stimulate saliva flow or else to sip on sweet liquids to wet the mouth. Don't do it! Increasing sugar consumption in the absence of saliva promotes disastrous tooth decay. If you want candy or gum, make sure it has xylitol. Xylitol is the one sweetener that actually inhibits cavity formation by constipating the acid-producing bacteria.

The first line of defense against dry mouth involves simple lifestyle changes. Start by limiting your intake of caffeine and alcohol. Both are natural diuretics—just ponder how quickly either one sends you to the bathroom. You may also have blessedly forgotten alcohol's strong association with "cotton mouth." Forego tobacco and marijuana, which both aggravate dry mouth symptoms.

If lifestyle changes don't solve the problem, you'll need other measures. Keep your mouth moist by drinking water frequently. Water beats any other liquid. because even sugar-free sodas are scarily acidic. Without saliva to neutralize the acid, drinking any kind of acidic beverage can erode your enamel.

Also try to keep your environment moist by running a humidifier if air is dry and breathing through your nose so you don't lose moisture through your mouth.

Over-the-counter saliva substitutes can also provide relief. You'll find a host of these spit-mimics on the drugstore shelves, but they provide temporary relief only. Dr. Susan's team prefers Biotene® moisturizing gel or CariFree® CTx2 spray. No matter which product you choose, look for the American Dental Association seal of approval and you can feel confident about using it.

Prescription saliva stimulants are generally indicated for patients with Sjögren's syndrome. But if your dry mouth is caused by medication, adding another medication to the mix, with additional side effects, might not be the best solution for the long run.

For maximum protection against tooth decay and enamel loss, dry mouth patients should get a professional fluoride varnish application every three months and use a concentrated at-home fluoride paste. To help strengthen enamel, add calcium phosphate application such as MI™ paste. One unique toothpaste that Dr. Susan recommends is CTx4 gel 1100 by CariFree™. This paste combines a therapeutic level of fluoride, calcium phosphate and xylitol in one paste. To order CTx4 gel 1100, talk to your dentist or check it out on CariFree.com.

To protect your mouth from cavities and gum disease, pay extra attention to daily home care. Remember that plaque you miss when brushing and flossing gets no cleansing help from your saliva.

Always alert your dentist if you develop dry mouth, and work with him or her to track down the cause and provide relief.

Quickstart to health

1. Work with your physician to change or eliminate medications that cause dry mouth.

If you take several medications, it may not be easy to identify the saliva-thief. Nor is it always possible to switch or eliminate medications prescribed for life-threatening problems. Better lifestyle choices, such as improved nutrition, regular exercise, more sleep and less stress can help eliminate conditions that require prescription medications.

2. Limit consumption of caffeine and alcohol, and avoid tobacco and street drugs.

Caffeine and alcohol are effective diuretics, and tobacco, marijuana and other recreational drugs are all notorious for producing dry mouth.

3. Keep your mouth moist by hydrating during the day.

Sip on water, suck on ice or on xylitol-sweetened candy, or chew xylitol-sweetened gum, such as Icebreakers or Trident.

4. Use an ADA-approved saliva substitute and/or consider a prescription for saliva stimulation.

Both over-the-counter substitutes and prescription saliva stimulants are available to help with your dry mouth. Ask your dentist, physician or pharmacist about the best options for you.

5. Keep your environment moist.

Use a humidifier to increase moisture in your home or office, especially in winter.

6. Breathe through your nose to keep as much moisture as possible in your mouth.

Brush your teeth with a toothpaste that contains fluoride as well as enamel protectors. Fluoride will protect your teeth from cavities, and ingredients such as calcium phosphate and Xylitol help strengthen and protect your enamel.

7. Get professional fluoride varnish applications every three months.

Fluoride works well to protect against enamel loss and tooth decay.

8. See your dentist regularly to protect your teeth and gums.

Visit your dentist at least twice a year for a protective examination and cleaning. Talk with her about your xerostomia and work together to establish a personalized tooth/gum protection plan.

SECTION 7

Psychological Health

WE'VE DISCUSSED HOW IMPROVED MOUTH HEALTH CAN HELP YOU lead a healthier, sexier life—but what about a happier one? It should be no surprise that your oral health also impacts your psychological health.

People with good oral health tend to smile more—and people who smile more are, quite simply, happier, as we discuss in Chapter 23, The Smile Bonus. They're also better positioned to lead successful lives. As an example, welfare recipients whose dental issues were treated didn't just enjoy better oral health; they also were more likely to get jobs and get off welfare.

Recent studies also show a relationship between a healthy mouth and Clinical Depression, as we explain in Chapter 24. It's long been known that many who suffer from long-lasting episodes of depression demonstrate a lapse in personal hygiene—including oral hygiene—at the same time. The result can often be rampant tooth decay and gum disease. But only recently have studies shown that poor oral health is actually a risk factor for depression.

Even if you don't suffer from depression and your mouth is in great shape, you may not feel as good about yourself as you could if you're not happy with your smile. If this is you, you may hide your teeth by trying not to smile too big or you may even cover your mouth with pinched lips or a raised hand. This can impact how happy you are and also how others think of you.

Cosmetic dentistry may be the answer. We discuss one of the simplest improvements in Chapter 25, Tooth Lightening. But other techniques, including orthodontics, bonding and veneers, can help you get closer to your ideal. Find out more about what's possible in Chapter 26, Tooth Alteration. And who knows? You may even smile more.

But all of this assumes you're comfortable visiting your dentist in the first place—and that's a stumbling block for millions of individuals with Dental Phobia, which we cover in Chapter 22. So many of you may need to start by finding a dental practice that understands your fears and works with you to manage the triggers.

Chapter 22

DENTAL PHOBIA: THE 2ND MOST FEARED CHAIR

RESEARCH CONTINUES TO SHOW THE IMPORTANCE of good oral health to your overall health. But there's one catch: You need to go see your dentist at least twice a year. That's a problem if you have dental anxiety, which afflicts about 75 percent of Americans. For some it's even worse: The American Dental Association estimates that 10 percent of Americans experience dental phobia so paralyzing that they avoid the dentist except when they suffer from pain or a major infection.

If we are talking about you, you now know that you are not alone. And who can blame you? The antiseptic smell, the shrill whine of the drill, the shot with the unusually long needle, the numbness that makes you wonder if you can even swallow, the claustrophobia when masked figures load up your mouth with fingers, spit suckers and cotton rolls, the feeling of being pinned down in the chair with no control over what happens next …

No wonder you freak out! But if you avoid the dental office at all costs, you can trigger a vicious cycle: Poor oral health that requires emergency and/or invasive treatment when you finally do see the dentist, further reinforcing your fear.

Much like post-traumatic stress disorder (PTSD), dental fear usually develops as a result of a disturbing dental experience, often during childhood. Such emotional trauma can occur in patients if they have ever suffered a painful, overbearing or frightening incident. That's heightened if the patient also felt a sense of helplessness or lack of control. In fact, any negative medical experience—or any history of physical, emotional or sexual abuse—can stimulate this dental "white coat syndrome."

After avoiding the dentist for longer than they should, these patients' dental anxiety is often heightened by the embarrassment of poor oral health and the fear of being ridiculed or scolded by the dentist.

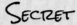

> ## SECRET
>
> Dental anxiety can be triggered by a smell or sound that unconsciously unlocks a bad memory and prompts a fight-or-flight response, even during routine visits. Talking with your dentist about how you can distract your brain and avoid triggers lets you receive preventive care, enjoy the advantages of good oral health—and by association, good overall health.

Taking control

If you have dental phobia, the relationship with your dentist becomes critical. Patients who have successfully overcome dental anxiety cite interpersonal factors that helped them. These include a dentist who gives thorough information and explanation, slows down the procedure, listens with empathy to their concerns and lets them control the treatment.

Dr. Susan finds that if she can put you, the patient, in control, the fear lessens. In her practice, she is willing to stop a procedure whenever a patient gives a pre-arranged signal. Because perceived pain is different for every person, she believes her patients should always have control over when to stop or go.

Identifying a dental practice, like Dr. Susan's, that helps you recognize and eliminate emotional triggers can also be helpful. Some dental teams use scents to change the smells typically associated with dentistry, wear non-traditional clinic attire or play music in the background—or give you headphones with your own choice of music to drown out the dental office sounds. Multi-sensory distraction that may be offered includes heat, light, sound, aromatherapy, therapeutic touch (such as a hand, foot or pressure-point massage) and vibration (such as a vibrating chair pad).

Treatments to manage fear

If you suffer from dental phobia, you may also want to consider targeted psychological treatments, such as eye movement desensitization and reprocessing (EMDR), a well-known therapy for PTSD. Cognitive behavioral therapy (CBT), a tool for managing stressful life situations, can also be helpful.

Dentists often use drugs in conjunction with behavioral techniques to help you manage dental fear. Those below—"laughing gas" (nitrous oxide) and drugs

ranging from mild prescription anti-anxiety meds to intravenous (IV) conscious
sedation—are most common.

Nitrous oxide or "laughing gas"

The beauties of nitrous are many. It is a mixture of two gases, nitrous oxide
(the relaxing drug) and straight oxygen. The strength can be turned up or down
depending on your level of anxiety. It's easy for a dentist to administer, requires
no prescription or trip to the drugstore, and spurs both relaxation and dissociation
without taking away your grasp of reality or your ability to communicate.

Nitrous is also easily offloaded. That means the effects go away completely
within five minutes of breathing straight oxygen, so you can drive home safely.
Dr. Susan notices that many dental phobics are also afraid of taking a drug that
would further interrupt their control over a situation. So the real bonus with
nitrous is that you can give it a try and change your mind in a few minutes if you
don't like the way you feel.

Anti-anxieties and sedatives

Oral anti-anxiety meds like Valium, Ativan or Xanax can also be useful. These
meds are generally taken in pill form just prior to the appointment. But in some
circumstances, IV conscious sedation is the answer. This "twilight sleep" lets
you respond to your dentist's prompts, but you may have little or no recollection
of the experience after a procedure. If you feel that you need this level of support
and your dentist isn't licensed and trained for IV sedation, ask him for a referral
to a well-qualified colleague.

Soothing your dental fear is critical to managing your oral health and your
overall health. By working with your dentist, you can develop a plan that will be
successful for you.

Quickstart to health

1. Understand that dental phobia usually arises from a traumatic event.

These events generally occur in childhood and often involve a bad dental experience or another invasion/trauma of the mouth or head and neck region.

2. Establish a relationship with an empathetic dentist.

Your dentist should provide thorough information about your procedure and let you choose how it progresses. You'll feel a lot more comfortable if you're in control.

3. Find a practice that alleviates emotional triggers.

Some dental teams work hard to offer a calming environment through smell, sight, temperature, sound and therapeutic touch. You may find these help distract your brain enough that you're not as fearful.

4. See a therapist for behavioral therapy.

Sometimes just distracting you from your fears isn't enough. A therapist can work with you to manage your PTSD and/or stress from life situations and trauma.

5. Talk with your dentist about anti-anxiety meds.

Dentists use a variety of drugs from laughing gas or oral anti-anxiety meds to IV sedation to ensure their patients enjoy calm, pain-free procedures.

Chapter 23
The Smile Bonus:
Happiness and Confidence

From the chair

MY PET-SITTER ALICIA *was a kind, sweet animal lover who adored my pup Ellie—and vice versa.*

But I couldn't help noticing her unsightly smile full of brown and broken teeth, an obvious result of rampant tooth decay. At only 32, she was embarrassed by her smile. She especially didn't smile at men her age. She dated occasionally, but men would rarely take her out in public with them. Other than pet-sitting, she was unemployed and relied on public transportation to get around town.

Alicia was what I call a sipper—she sipped on Mountain Dew all day long. Like many people, she didn't really believe her bad teeth were associated with her soda-sipping habit. But after her first educational visit with my dental team, she kicked the habit cold. Not surprisingly, she immediately began to lose weight.

Over the next four months, my team restored her smile to one she could be proud to flash. When she finally saw her bright, beautiful teeth in the mirror for the first time, tears filled her eyes and started trickling down her cheeks.

But the real transformation happened after that. Within the next year, Alicia blossomed into a great big smiler who was 60 pounds lighter. She had interviewed and was hired for a fulltime position as a customer service representative, bought a car, fell in love with her "prince" and began house hunting with her husband-to-be.

Is this all a result of a new smile? Alicia says so: "Sugar is evil! It's amazing how having beautiful teeth improves your life."

As it turns out, there's ample research to support her notion.

> ## Secret
>
> Smiling makes you happier, even if you didn't smile because you're happy. And being happy produces a laundry list of healthy effects, from lower blood pressure to higher self-esteem.

Smile your way to happiness

When you're happy, you probably engage in the same behavior as most of us: You smile.

That comes as no surprise. But you may not realize this behavior also works in reverse: If you smile, you'll be happier. As Vietnamese Zen Master Thich Nhat Hanh says, "Sometimes your joy is the source of your smile, but sometimes your smile can be the source of your joy."

Studies have shown that just engaging the smile muscles—especially the *zygomaticus major*—releases endorphins in our brains. Even *faking* a smile releases tiny spurts of the stuff that makes us feel better.

In a 1988 study led by Fritz Strack of the University of Würzberg in Germany, a group of participants were asked to hold a pencil in their lips. A second group of participants were asked to hold the pencil in their teeth—with their lips not touching, thereby engaging their smile muscles. This second group, the unknowing "smilers," ranked the comics they were viewing as significantly funnier than the straight-lipped group.

Wait, there's more. Smiles are also contagious—they make other people inadvertently smile and feel happier, which in turn influences a more positive response toward *you*. And yes, the opposite is also true: Frowning also triggers others to unconsciously frown and, in turn, feel worse.

These emotional contagions are a result of an inherent physiologic process called *mimicry*. Our ancestors' abilities to empathize with or "danger-warn" by mimicking their neighbors' emotions were sometimes the communication determinants between life and death.

So how much better does smiling make you feel? Research has shown that smiling has measurable elevating effects on the body: It boosts our immune system, reduces stress, lowers blood pressure, enhances others' perceptions of us and, as you've probably noticed, significantly improves our impact.

Authentic smiles are also marked by engagement of an eye muscle called the *obicularis oculii*. So don't worry if you have crow's feet—squinty, smiley eyes convey and spread feelings of amusement, optimism and joy.

Smile your way to self-esteem

As part of her cosmetic dentistry practice, Dr. Susan performs smile makeovers, which often include both functional and aesthetic aspects. But often she finds that, like Alicia, far more than her patient's smile improves after the procedure.

Her team has been particularly curious about the psychological impact of smile makeovers. They expected the "before" and "after" photos to show an amazing difference, but they didn't necessarily expect the "before" and "after" lives to show such improvement.

As Dr. Susan notes:

I have watched many adults just like Alicia dramatically change their life circumstances in the year or two that follows a smile makeover. It seems the profound boost of confidence gives people courage to get a promotion, improve personal relationships, achieve better nutrition and fitness, and increase their personal energy.

That may be particularly true in the United States, where we place a high value on an aesthetically pleasing smile. Brighter, straighter, stronger looking teeth are a symbol of health and success.

Not surprisingly then, Dr. Susan has found that a person who has small, discolored, crowded or misshapen teeth often becomes self-conscious of their smile during adolescence. These kids learn early how to hide their teeth, either with their lips or hands. As you learned previously, smiling even when you're not happy can make you feel better. So imagine the impact of constantly trying not to smile.

What might happen when you reverse that? First you'd experience a boost of natural endorphins the first time you flashed a full-blown smile after years of hiding it.

Second you'd find your big, bright smile is irresistible to others—even strangers might feel drawn to smile back. So imagine how much friendlier the world would seem when at last you could show warmth and good humor to everyone around you.

As others responded more positively to you, your confidence would climb. Suddenly you might find yourself taking risks you've only dreamed of: asking for a promotion or a date, or giving a front-of-the-room presentation. Or even, like Alicia, getting your first real job.

In a 2006 study co-authored by Dr. Susan Hyde, a dentist and population scientist at the University of California, San Francisco, the researchers offered treatments to 377 welfare recipients with severe dental problems—including seriously receding gums and missing or decaying teeth. Following dental treatment, 79 percent showed better oral-health-related quality-of-life scores. But in addition, those who completed the treatment were twice as likely to move off welfare or get jobs than those who didn't.

Dr. Susan's team has also noted how often enhancing a patient's smile inspires other health changes, such as improved fitness, nutrition or energy. Often they quit smoking or improve personal and oral hygiene.

If you've read *The Power of Habit* by Charles Duhigg, you're aware that changing some habits can be a powerful force, because they create a chain reaction. As you adopt these "keystone" habits, you'll notice they trickle down into other areas of your life. For example, you may start to exercise and find that you've improved your diet as well.

Likewise a healthy, beautiful smile can not only have a profound impact on your happiness and self-esteem, but it can also be the trigger that changes other aspects of your life and encourages new habits that improve your life.

Quickstart to health

1. Brush and floss to make sure your smile looks as good as it can.

The first step is always good oral hygiene to maximize the health and appearance of your teeth and gums. There's no question that beautiful begins with healthy.

2. Treat any oral health issues immediately.

Discolorations on teeth, red or purplish gums, shifting/drifting teeth, chipping/cracking teeth—these may all be warning signs of oral health problems such as tooth decay, gum disease, grinding or acid erosion. See your dentist to take care of problems and improve function and aesthetics.

3. Consider improvements to the aesthetics of your teeth and gums if you're hiding your smile.

A number of treatments have been designed to give you a bright, beautiful smile without a major investment in cosmetic dentistry. For example, teeth lightening can brighten dull, yellow teeth; composite bonding, veneers or crowns can repair chipped, broken, poorly shaped teeth; and tooth-colored or invisible braces can straighten teeth almost imperceptibly.

4. Consult your dentist if you believe your current smile is keeping you from a happy, full life.

Depending on the current state of your teeth and the look you'd like to achieve, you may decide on a complete smile makeover. This can make the largest difference in the aesthetics of your mouth and in your happiness and self-esteem.

Chapter 24

Clinical Depression and Oral Health: A Two-Way Street

In May 2014, a group of researchers at the Deakin IMPACT Strategic Research Centre in Australia reported on a connection they'd found between poor dental health and depression. What they discovered flipped what's known about the relationship between the two on its head—and spurred new questions about cause and effect.

Clinical depression is a psychiatric illness that impairs mood, thoughts and behavioral patterns, and lasts at least two weeks. The illness causes enormous distress and impairs an individual's social functioning and quality of life.

Symptoms include prolonged sadness, hopelessness and irritability, loss of interest in favorite activities, withdrawal from people, changes in sleep patterns, weight gain or loss, and diminished self-care, including personal hygiene.

These symptoms impact millions of us. In a given year, some 14.8 million American adults are stricken with a major depressive order, according to the Depression and Bipolar Support Alliance. Over the course of a lifetime, women experience depression at about twice the rate of men. The incidence is 20 percent to 26 percent for women and 8 percent to 12 percent for men.

Depression often goes undiagnosed, untreated and unmentioned, although the death rate is higher than that for breast cancer. In part that's because our society still views mental illness as a character weakness, not as an imbalance in brain chemistry. The personal shame that results often serves as a barrier against getting help.

Studies indicate that the most effective treatment today is a combination of antidepressants *and* cognitive behavior therapy, in which the patient learns to think differently about his circumstances.

How depression impacts dental health

Depression impacts oral health in a variety of ways, all negative. The associated lack of interest in personal hygiene means those suffering from depression often go a week, two weeks or even longer with little care for their teeth.

If you don't interrupt plaque with a brush and floss on a regular basis—and by that, we mean every 24 hours—the bacterial makeup of the plaque gets scarier by the day. Depending on your age and general health, this can put you at high risk for periodontal disease and active infection. People with depression often smoke more, which certainly worsens gum disease.

At the same time the bacterial load is increasing, saliva flow may be decreasing as a side effect of antidepressants. That boosts the risk of tooth decay. Add a soda-sipping habit or a growing taste for carbs as serotonin levels plummet, and rampant decay could be the result. The coupling of gum disease and tooth decay can also lead to horrific bad breath, which can repulse family and friends.

The additional stress brought on by depression also compromises the immune system and speeds up the breakdown of gums and supporting bone. Medications for stress and depression can both stimulate clenching and grinding, causing worn or broken teeth, debilitating headaches, and facial or temporomandibular joint pain.

How dental health impacts depression

Is there any good news? Not really—but there is new news. For decades or longer, researchers have known about the undesirable impacts we just discussed. But only recently did they ask whether poor dental health also increases the likelihood of depression.

In the study by the Deakin IMPACT Strategic Research Centre, the investigators measured dental health by the number of dental conditions a subject had. They gathered the data from the U.S. National Health and Nutrition Examination Surveys (NHANES 2005-2008).

The study found that the incidence of depression was greater for those who suffered from more dental conditions. But even more interesting, the researchers found a dose-response relationship: The more dental conditions a subject had, the greater the severity of their depression. The researchers controlled for known contributing factors in depression, including a marker for inflammation (the C-reactive protein) and body mass index.

Depression is considered an inflammatory disorder, so sources of inflammation in the body caused by other factors can contribute to mental disorders. Dental diseases such as periodontitis increase inflammation in the body and have been linked with a number of systemic diseases. But only recently have researchers looked at the connections with mental health.

At the 43rd Annual Meeting & Exhibition of the American Association for Dental Research, R. Constance Wiener, Ph.D., from West Virginia University, presented data from a telephone survey of more than 77,000 respondents. The data showed that depression, anxiety and a combination of the two are also associated with tooth loss.

Although both studies discussed here found a link between clinical depression and poor dental health, as yet the relationship is not well-understood. But the results confirm the importance of oral health and bacteria on both physical and mental diseases with inflammatory origins.

Quickstart to health

1. Don't be ashamed.

Just as periodontitis results from inflammation of your gums, depression may result from an inflammation in your brain—not a fault in your brain itself. If you're depressed, talk about your symptoms with trusted friends and medical professionals.

2. Seek professional help.

Speak with your physician about a strategy for help or a referral to a specialist. The best results may be achieved through a combination of therapy and drugs.

3. Consider counseling or cognitive therapy.

Ask your physician for a referral. Cognitive therapy, for example, may help you to change negative thought patterns and improve how you feel about your circumstances.

4. Consider antidepressant medication.

Many drugs offer short-term or long-term relief from depression. This is especially important if your relationships are in danger and critical if you've thought of harming yourself.

5. Eat a good diet.

When levels of feel-good chemicals like serotonin drop, the urge to load up on carbs and junk food increases. Try to focus on good nutrition, including lean protein and lots of fruits and vegetables.

6. Exercise at least 10 minutes a day.

If you can commit to 10 minutes, chances are you'll decide you can keep going for 15, 20 or even 30 minutes. That's good, because exercise increases serotonin levels and helps you sleep—and in a vicious cycle, missing sleep can make it hard to climb out of depression.

A call to action: Talk about depression openly. The more we normalize this disease, the better off we ALL are. If this discussion reminds you of someone you love, have the courage to begin a conversation about depression. You may just be saving a life.

Chapter 25

Tooth Lightening: The Secret to Pearly Whites

ALMOST EVERYONE AGREES THAT A SMILE is an important social asset, one that makes you more approachable to new friends, increases your sex appeal and gives you a noted advantage when you compete for a promotion or work to close a sale. When Dr. Susan asks her patients what it would take for them to feel better about their smiles, they almost always start with this: "I'd like my teeth to be whiter and brighter."

Bright, white teeth are a symbol of youth. In fact, our first set of teeth, the baby teeth, are generally sparkly white. Parents can be undone when they notice that their children's permanent teeth come in somewhat darker. If you assume you're looking at a surface layer of stain, you might even send your kids back to the bathroom to brush better. But that rarely helps.

Tooth shades are mostly influenced by the *inner* layer of tooth structure, called the dentin. Genetics determine much of natural tooth shade, so without other influencing factors, the shade is what you inherit. That's true until you see signs of age-related discoloration—which is what most of us object to when we look in the mirror. The onset and rate of that yellowing varies from person to person. Fortunately we can now turn back time.

> **Secret**
>
> Tooth lightening can brighten your teeth and make you more comfortable with your smile. But chasing an unceasing glow-in-the-dark smile can damage pulp and cause teeth to die an untimely death.

The causes of discoloration

Factors other than age can discolor teeth as well. Some people have surface stains from drinking dark beverages like red wine and coffee, eating foods like blueberries and tomato sauce, and smoking or chewing tobacco. Your dental hygienist or dentist can readily remove these stains. Whitening toothpastes can also handle changes in tooth color due to stains. These pastes contain polishing and chemical agents to remove surface stain but don't contain peroxide-like bleaching agents. If you choose a whitening toothpaste, make sure it has the ADA Seal of Acceptance. To learn more about what's in toothpaste, see Chapter 35, Your Toothpaste.

Internal discoloration of a natural tooth can be caused by aging but also from a developmental defect, antibiotics (such as tetracycline) taken during childhood, decay, old silver/black fillings that tarnish the enamel from the inside of the tooth, or tooth trauma, such as a blow to the mouth, which causes the nerve and blood supply to die.

To brighten a dark tooth, Dr. Susan will replace a dark filling or sometimes bleach the tooth from a chamber drilled into the back of it. If these fail to do the trick, she will restore the outside of the tooth with a whiter covering, such as composite bonding, a porcelain veneer or crown.

The Hollywood smile

Most people don't want to lighten just one discolored tooth; they want to whiten and brighten *all* their teeth. For that dentists use peroxide-containing bleaching agents applied to the outside of the teeth. The peroxide percolates right through the glass-like tubules that make up the enamel to lighten the inner dentin layer.

Over the years, manufacturers have developed a number of ways to bleach teeth. Most are safe, but some are more effective than others. Several over-the-counter products, such as Crest Whitestrips, paints or self-molded trays, are available and many are helpful, especially if your teeth are straight and you are not seeking a dramatic improvement.

The state of the art for lightening is still constructing custom-fitted trays made from a mold or model of your teeth and applied under the guidance of your dentist. To use these individually designed, clear-plastic flexible trays, you dab bleaching gel into the small receptacles for each tooth. This works best if you wear the trays for a minimum of four to six hours, so usually dentists recommend bedtime use.

In-office one-hour lightening does give you a jumpstart on the process, but some of the initial lightening is actually from dehydration and doesn't last. In-office lightening is almost always followed by tray lightening, which does most of the work. That jumpstart comes at a price: The cost is usually twice as much as custom tray lightening. Note also that if your dentist suggests laser or light activation as a significant enhancement to in-office bleaching procedures, just say "No." Research does not show that it increases effectiveness.

The issues

If it seems too good to be true, it may still be true—but it may come with side effects. In the case of bleaching, peroxide-based products may cause temporary temperature sensitivity and sometimes gum irritation. You must use the bleaching gel as directed and let your dentist determine the appropriate concentration (usually 10 percent to 20 percent) of the carbamide peroxide. For significant sensitivity, Dr. Susan recommends slowing down the bleaching process, decreasing the bleach concentration and treating the teeth with fluoride and/or other desensitizers during the process.

Once your teeth have reached the level of brightness you desire, you can store your trays until they're needed again. Although whitening does not wear off, your teeth will continue to drift at the same age-discoloring rate as before. In a year or two, you may want to lighten again for a few more nights. If so, you'll probably need to buy more bleach, because it loses its *oomph* over time. Check the expiration date and store bleach in the fridge to get the most shelf life you can.

Also note that bleaching works only on natural tooth structure, not on existing crowns or fillings. After you whiten you will likely notice that old fillings stand out. So when you're determining the cost of bleaching, you may want to add in the fees for replacing old fillings with tooth-colored materials.

One final word of caution: You should not bleach continually. Dr. Susan has encountered patients who become addicted to bleaching—always chasing down the glow-in-the-dark smile that can't be sustained. This, like any other addiction, poses physical dangers such as pulpal damage, otherwise known as tooth death.

The price of perfection

The cost of bleaching with custom trays doesn't come cheap—but it is a long-term investment. When you need to bleach again, you can just pull out your trays and buy a refill tube of bleach at a minimal cost.

Initially the cost of white strips will be less, but if you buy a box every year or two, the cost will add up. So it will be more expensive in the long run.

Dr. Susan notices that women balk far less at the $500+ cost for professional bleaching than men do. Add up what most women spend on hair, makeup, clothing and jewelry in a year, and the investment in white teeth is a steal. And there's no denying that a bright smile looks good with everything.

Quickstart to health

1. Start with healthy teeth and gums.

Make sure all surface stains and plaque or tartar have been professionally removed from your teeth before lightening. Treat any tooth decay and gum disease before spending money on cosmetics. Again, healthy is beautiful.

2. For modest changes, try over-the-counter products.

For straight-ish teeth that need only a shade or two of lightening, try Crest Whitestrips. This might be enough for you to achieve the results you want.

3. See your dentist for more dramatic lightening.

Invest in custom-fitted bleach trays and use only professionally dispensed bleach products such as carbamide peroxide in 10 percent or 15 percent concentrations.

4. Manage sensitivity with the help of your dentist.

Let your dentist guide you and monitor your progress and sensitivity. Desensitizing strategies vary, but sensitivity from lightening is almost always temporary.

5. Store custom bleach trays for later use.

After achieving your ideal shade, store your bleach trays for use in a year or so. When you're ready, repurchase a new batch of bleach gel from your dentist.

Chapter 26

TOOTH ALTERATION: CREATING BEAUTY

From the chair

I WENT HEAD TO HEAD WITH SHELIA, *a 24-year-old beauty, over her decision to keep her mouth jewelry—a silver-balled tongue piercing that had already chipped three cusps off her back teeth. When I called it "the wrecking ball," Shelia was obviously taken aback. So I took a step back too and re-engaged with total curiosity:*

"I'm so sorry if I have offended you, Shelia. You see, I'm a self-proclaimed tooth geek, in the tooth-saving business. I am really curious to know why you are so attached to keeping that thing that is mutilating your teeth."

Shelia answered in five simple words: "Cuz it looks so cool."

Shelia was speaking for an entire globe of adults when she replied with such honesty. We don't only use our mouth for chewing and speaking; we also use it to attract others. But our ideas about beauty differ across cultures and even generations within a culture.

If you've ever studied dental anthropology, you might know that in the pre-classic era (100 B.C.-300 A.D.), Mesoamerican artisans would painstakingly (pun intended) inlay jewels, such as turquoise, jade or gold, into the surfaces of teeth. In fact, in some cultures, mutilation of teeth was viewed as a sign of social status. A rite of passage among the young Moi of Vietnam, for example, involved chipping the front teeth and grinding them down to the gumline to create beauty. Youngsters who refused were considered neither grown-up nor marriageable.

For us in America, these practices seem entirely strange, because we take for granted our own ideals. So what do we hold as our ideal of dental beauty? We prefer teeth that are white, perfectly positioned, straight up and down, and symmetric from one side to the other. Movie stars, models and others in the limelight know that we indirectly associate straight, white teeth with health, vigor and youth, and are willing to have their teeth "fixed" to achieve the ideal.

And they're not alone. The concept of smile makeovers grew like wildfire from 2002 to 2007, when CBS's "Extreme Makeover" show streamed into millions of living rooms. To Dr. Susan, it seemed that of all the miracles on the show, the smile makeover was the most impressive—to say nothing of the longest lasting. And often it did the most to boost the individual's self-confidence.

Dentists across the country got busy studying "smile design" and changing their street signs to read "cosmetic dentist." This media boost plus innovative materials equaled a cosmetic dentistry explosion. Many men and women tired of hiding their smiles decided "I'll put my money where my mouth is," even if it was just for a brighter and whiter smile.

You can learn more about that option in Chapter 25, Tooth Lightening. But what other techniques help us achieve our ideal smile?

Orthodontics

Kids wearing braces seems like an American rite of passage, with estimates that 50 percent to 70 percent of youngsters will experience "ortho" sometime between 6 and 18 years of age. Moving teeth with hardware is not a new concept—in fact, as early as 1728, a famous dentist named Pierre Fauchard used a "bandeau," a horseshoe-shaped piece of metal, to expand the arch.

As kids, Dr. Susan and Diana were both "metal mouths": Each wore wall-to-wall metal bands around each one of their teeth. But by the mid-1970s, the age of bonding adhesives arrived and ortho changed forever. By bonding brackets directly on the face of a tooth, fewer extractions were necessary. Kids ended up with bigger, broader smiles, but they weren't the only ones to benefit. Adults started wearing braces too, especially if they missed out as youngsters.

The biggest deterrent for adults, however, was the appearance of the braces themselves. In 1996, 3-D computer imaging collided with the field of orthodontics—and by the early 2000s, Invisalign® (invisible braces) and short-term ortho for adults had arrived. Today the most widely recognized system of short-term braces is Six Month Smiles, which uses clear brackets and white wires to blend with the teeth. The treatment focuses on using the back teeth for stability and moving front teeth into better alignment, so it takes less time.

Adults deserve straight teeth too, but one of Dr. Susan's esteemed teachers, Dr. Vince Kocich, said it this way: "Kids ought to be treated ideally and adults, realistically." Not every patient is a candidate for fast movement—this depends on the health of the supporting gums and bone, temporomandibular joint (TMJ) stability and skeletal structure.

In Dr. Susan's opinion, ortho cases that use fast movement don't always finish with ideal bite relationships. If you're considering this option, make sure your dentist is equally concerned about finishing the case with attention to stabilizing your bite, TMJs and long-term tooth alignment.

> ## Secret
> Patients feel guilty that their straightening "relapses," because they didn't wear retainers long enough. But the best retainer is teeth that fit together with equal and opposing forces—and in harmony with healthy TMJ positions. A stable bite will pay off in the long run with healthier teeth, bones and TMJs.

What does the future of ortho hold? Cutting-edge, high-tech systems use a 3-D scanned image of your teeth to help the orthodontist plan for a precise treatment outcome. Once the blueprint is established, systems like *SureSmile* use a highly accurate robot to customize the series of arch wires needed for treatment. This shortens the treatment time and gives highly accurate results. With new developments, we can expect braces to be smaller, less visible, more comfortable, worn for shorter periods and to produce more accurate outcomes.

Bonding

When Dr. Susan graduated from dental school in 1985, it was still considered taboo to remove enamel for any reason other than to treat disease. So if you did remove enamel, it was only to prepare for a filling, crown, tooth implant or bridge.

Before "bonding," dentists used white glasslike materials to fill front teeth, instead of silver or gold. The fillings were not color-stable for very long and didn't really bond to the tooth, so decay often recurred.

But then came adhesion dentistry—and the ability to stick anything to anything for a long time. That included building a chemical bond by acid-etching a tooth and painting it with a new kind of glue that would seal the enamel to the composite. But the material scientists didn't stop there.

Their next big innovation let dentists bond the dentin—the inner layer of tooth structure—to the composite. Add curing lights and now dentists could play around with the material until it was ready to set, then zap it with UV light to harden it.

Veneers

Next came composite veneers, which became popular in the 1980s. Dentists were able to bond over a tooth with a sculpted layer of tooth-looking material—an illusion of straight, white teeth. Today dentists have access to gorgeous composite materials. Those with skilled and artistic hands can create lifelike smiles in a single visit.

More popular is the ceramic veneer, a thin, laboratory-made, glass-like shell that dentists bond onto the tooth—a single tooth to hide a fracture or flaw, or a whole grill of teeth for a Hollywood smile. These veneers last for 10 to 30 years and, if done well, can create a huge boost in self-confidence.

One downside is they almost always require some tooth drilling to shape the tooth to receive the veneer. Your mind might now be drifting back toward the beginning of the chapter, to what a cultural anthropologist might label as "mutilation for beauty." And it's true that over-preparation of teeth can result in trauma, from temporary cold sensitivity to pulp death. If you are considering veneers to "correct" significant tooth crowding, an advanced restorative dentist might suggest orthodontic straightening, even for four to eight months, to reduce the amount of tooth trimming needed for veneers.

Veneers today are made of the same tooth-mimicking material as "aesthetic" crowns. Veneers, also called laminates, are bonded to the front of the tooth, whereas crowns encompass the whole tooth and are designed for structural support, not just for beauty.

The most recent advances in veneers rely on 3-D computer-aided design and machining technology. Dentists can now design a single tooth or your whole smile in virtual reality and have the computer transmit that design information to a desktop milling station. The mill begins with small blocks of zirconia and spits out your veneer or crown in minutes—with no temporaries. But in Dr. Susan's opinion, the final outcome is not yet as lifelike and magical as hand-layered porcelain built by a skilled ceramic artist.

> " **SECRET**
>
> If you are having your teeth restored with crowns or veneers due to wear, have a plan to control continued wear before you rebuild. Porcelain or zirconia can wear down or fracture opposing teeth even more than enamel. Work with your dentist to fix your occlusion or make a plan to protect your teeth, your self-esteem and your wallet. "

Eye of the beholder

Whether you're considering veneers, crowns or even a removable denture that re-designs your smile—the front of your face—it's a major change in how you see yourself and how others see you.

The smile makeover might begin with pictures you like that your dentist translates into a study model blueprint called a diagnostic wax-up. The wax-up is converted to a temporary or provisional smile for you to test-drive and poll your closest friends. After your dentist reshapes your provisional to meet your preferences, the prototype is communicated to the ceramic artist. The artist will use layers of glass-like sculpture to mimic the shape, length, contours and alignment of your smile to ensure a stunning outcome.

It's true—beauty is in the eye of the beholder—and you are the ultimate beholder. So no matter what treatment you are considering to beautify your smile, make sure your dentist wants to work *with* you, not *on* you—and that she listens and responds to your ideas about the outcome you desire.

Quickstart to health

1. Consult your dentist.

If your self-confidence is low because you are ashamed of your smile, ask your dentist for ideas. If he doesn't offer ideas that feel right for you, ask for a referral to an accomplished cosmetic dentist.

2. Be an advocate for function as well as beauty.

Make sure your orthodontist will consider more than looks. He should also focus on attaining a stable bite relationship in harmony with your TMJs.

3. Consider a combination of treatments.

If your teeth are super crowded or poorly positioned, consider orthodontic alignment before veneers or crowns. Less tooth reduction means less trauma to the pulp plus more overall biomechanical strength.

4. Insist on collaboration.

No matter how acclaimed your cosmetic dentist is, your perceptions about tooth lengths, contours, alignment and color should matter at least as much as the dentist's or dental laboratory technicians' preferences.

SECTION 8

Sexual Health and Satisfaction

IN ALMOST ALL CULTURES, nose-rubbing Eskimos aside, the mouth plays a starring role in mating. But it can also provide important clues about the status of your sexual health and satisfaction. In this section, we'll look at some of the key issues, from the deadly impact of oral cancer to the frustration of erectile dysfunction to the seemingly benign annoyance of snoring.

In 2010, veteran actor Michael Douglas shocked his fans, friends, publicist and perhaps his wife when he told the media that he was recovering from oral cancer—and suggested that the disease was caused by human papillomavirus (HPV) he had contracted while performing oral sex. In Chapter 27, Oral Cancer, we'll tell you the rest of the story, including how HPV infection has contributed to the growing incidence of oral cancer, especially among young non-smokers.

Chapter 28 discusses the recent report of a link between Erectile Dysfunction and periodontitis. A Turkish study found that men with gum disease are 3.3 times more likely to have erectile dysfunction. That may be the best incentive yet for men to get serious about brushing and flossing.

Prevention also figures in Chapter 29, Chapped Lips. Most of us treat chapped lips with balm after the fact, instead of protecting our lips from damage caused by the environment and especially sun exposure. That can be a serious lapse, given the potential for squamous cell carcinoma, a common form of skin cancer.

Chapter 30, Bad Breath, focuses on an issue you may regard as frivolous—but how serious it is depends on the kind of bad breath you have. If last night's garlic pesto is at fault, you may have nothing to worry about. But long-lasting bad breath can be a sign of serious disease—to say nothing of the damper it can put on your romantic life.

Chapter 31, Mouth Sores, discusses the most common kinds—only one of which is related to sex. But none of them will improve your sex appeal. We'll answer the three questions patients most frequently ask: Which sore do I have? What caused it? And what can I do to get rid of it … fast?

Chapter 32 wraps up this section with a look at Snoring. In a recent survey by the American Academy of Dental Sleep Medicine, 39 percent of respondents said snoring in the opposite sex is a turn-off. The #1 reaction in bed partners—presumably while they're lying awake with little else to do—is to worry about the snorer's health. That's a reasonable concern given the link between snoring and chronic diseases ranging from diabetes to high blood pressure to heart disease.

Chapter 27

Oral Cancer: From Love and Other Drugs

In late 2009, veteran actor Michael Douglas experienced a painfully sore tooth. He suspected he had a serious infection with the kind of gut-wrenching pain that could bring even *Wall Street* villain Gordon Gekko to his knees.

Nine months later, after one round after another of antibiotics that did nothing to stop the pain, a Montreal specialist examined Douglas' mouth. What he found was a walnut-sized tumor at the base of Douglas' tongue that no other physician had seen. The specialist ordered a biopsy.

Just as Douglas started touring to promote 2010's *Wall Street: Money Never Sleeps*, the actor came forward with his diagnosis—throat cancer.

The blight of oral cancer

The throat cancer Douglas experienced falls under the general category of oral cancer. Oral cancer can make you unable to swallow or chew, subject you to severe disfigurement from surgery to remove tumors and kill you if not caught early enough.

So Douglas inspired our sympathy with his diagnosis and then our curiosity when he later said his cancer was caused by the human papillomavirus (HPV), which can be contracted through oral sex.

Douglas' spokesman was quick to deny the link, insisting that what Douglas meant to say is that oral sex can cause certain oral cancers but was not necessarily the root of Douglas' own disease.

And in fact, Douglas has also drank and smoked for years, both known causes of oral cancer. Before the emergence of HPV, smoking was the #1 risk factor for oral cancer, made worse when combined with regular alcohol consumption.

But Douglas had it right—because his disease, which was ultimately revealed to be tongue cancer, occurred at the back of his mouth. That's where oral cancers related to HPV occur. Those caused by smoking and drinking are more often found on the floor of the mouth or sides of the tongue.

The good news for Douglas: When caught early enough, HPV-related cancers are more responsive to radiation and chemotherapy than other oral cancers.

Douglas underwent intense treatment and was given the all-clear in early 2011. But he went a step further: To warn others of the health risks of HPV, he donated his time and skills to create a public service announcement for the Oral Cancer Foundation.

We applaud Douglas for bravely bringing to light a link that many remain unaware of—the link between oral sex and increased risk of mouth cancer.

> ## Secret
>
> Among newly diagnosed cases of oral cancer, the fastest-growing segment is people under 40 infected with HPV type-16. Vaccination lowers the risk of acquiring HPV and of oral cancer.

The new oral cancer patient: The under-40 set

The risk of oral cancer does not increase simply from having sex but rather from transmission of certain high-risk types of HPV through intimate contact. HPV is one of the most common virus groups in the world and appears in many guises.

How common is HPV? According to the Centers for Disease Control and Prevention (CDC), 20 million Americans are currently infected. Another 6 million are newly infected each year.

The acronym HPV is actually a catch-all representing 120 known types of the virus. The low-risk types cause skin lesions, such as warts. The high-risk types, such as HPV-16 and HPV-18, are linked to approximately 70 percent of cervical cancers in women. But recent studies show these same high-risk types of HPV, along with HPV-6 and HPV-10, cause approximately 60 percent of cancers in the mouth, including those on the tonsils, throat and back of the tongue, according to *Lancet Oncology*.

HPV-type 16 poses the highest risk for oral cancers—up to 32 times more susceptibility, depending on the viral count.

Did you gloss over that? Read it again. That statistic says that the risk of developing oral cancer from HPV-16 could be more than 10 times the risk of developing it from smoking (three times the risk) or habitual alcohol use (two times the risk). So here's a special note for teens and sexually active adults: No matter what you've heard, there is no safe sex—not even oral sex.

The American Cancer Society estimates that in 2015, 39,500 people will be diagnosed with oral cancer and 7,500 will die from it. A study conducted in Saõ Paulo, Brazil, showed that among newly diagnosed cases, the fastest-growing segment is individuals under 40 years old. They need not be smokers or drinkers.

Most startling is the fact that although many other cancers have been in decline in recent years, the occurrence of oral cancers has increased each of the last six years. In fact, the numbers of HPV-related oral cancers will surpass cervical cancers in the near future.

Vaccines currently target the four most threatening types of HPV but will soon be reformulated to include four more. Even without vaccination, our body's natural immune system works to "clear" HPV so that it's no longer detectable within 12 to 18 months of infection. That sounds positive, but it doesn't work for everyone. If your body can't clear the virus, you carry a *persistent* HPV infection—making you more susceptible to cancer. You'll need frequent and thorough professional oral cancer screenings.

Critical diagnosis

How would you know if you have a persistent HPV infection? The good and bad news is that HPV infections have no telling signs or symptoms in the mouth. But a simple, professional swish, gargle and spit test administered in your dental office can give you the answer. The test, called OraRisk™, is analyzed by OralDNA Labs and can detect HPV infection in the early stages and identify 51 different types, including the 25 types that have been identified in oral cancer.

If you test positive for *any* of these, you should repeat the test 12 months later. If you still test positive, your dentist and perhaps an oral surgeon or ear, nose and throat specialist will partner with you to aggressively screen for, and remove, any potential pre-cancerous or cancerous lesions. The only way to truly diagnose cancer is by looking at the biopsy sample cells through a microscope.

That's critical, because if we find these cancers early, the survival rate is approximately 83 percent, according to the American Cancer Society. But at this time, two-thirds of oral cancers are found as late-stage, advanced cancers. This accounts, in part, for the high death rate: 5- and 10-year survival rates are 62 percent and 51 percent, respectively. Death rates from other cancers have declined as people get annual checks for the disease—and this could be true for oral cancer as well. All that's needed is simple, painless screening as part of routine dental and physical exams.

Not off the hook: Smokers and drinkers

So should smokers and drinkers breathe easily? Hardly. Smoking and drinking pack a double whammy: They put you at greater risk for HPV and for the hardest-to-treat non-HPV related cancers.

A recent Johns Hopkins study reported in *JAMA* showed that HPV-16 infection is more common among people who have recently used or been exposed to tobacco, regardless of their sexual behavior. The researchers theorized that perhaps tobacco users have a harder time clearing the virus from their bodies.

Heavy drinkers might want to reevaluate their habits too. According to a recent study by Moffitt Cancer Center in the journal *Sexually Transmitted Infections*, men who consume more alcohol also have a greater risk of HPV infection—independent of how many sexual partners they've had.

> ## Secret
>
> Alcohol inhibits our immune responses, causing increasing susceptibility to both bacterial and viral infections like HPV. To keep your immune system healthy, limit alcohol to two drinks a day if you're a man and one drink a day if you're a woman.

The price of prevention

To lower the risk of cervical and penile cancer, the CDC recommends vaccination against HPV at the age of 11 or 12. Three shots of Gardasil® or Cervarix® over six months protect against HPV infection. This may give us a false sense of security, however, because we don't yet know when the protection drops off and if re-vaccination will be as effective.

The vaccine is available and covered by health insurance only until the age of 21 in boys and 26 in girls. The suggestion is that this is for public health reasons. The thinking: By those ages, young men and women have likely been exposed, so we should save the vaccine for someone who can benefit from it.

We don't agree. After all, finding cervical cancer from a "preventive" pap smear or oral cancer from an oral cancer "screening" exam is not truly preventive, is it? Certainly it's not preventive like vaccination. We need more research on the potential benefits of vaccinating older men and women who haven't been exposed to or who have cleared HPV.

Contrary to what you may have heard, if you are beyond the covered benefit age for vaccination, you can still act as your own health advocate. If you're willing to spend $200 to $300 out of pocket, you can get vaccinated by walking into your local pharmacy.

Quickstart to health

1. Find out if you're infected with HPV.

Ask your dentist for an HPV-16 saliva test. It's as easy as swishing with saline and spitting in a cup. If you're positive for any of the types, retest in a year to see if the virus is cleared or persistent.

2. Make sure your dentist performs a complete oral cancer screening.

During your regular dental visit, your dentist will look for lumps, bumps, and asymmetric areas in your head and neck as well as abnormal patches in your mouth, sores and other abnormalities. Oral cancer can be any color: red, black, brown or even normal flesh, so you cannot easily identify it yourself.

3. If you have a persistent HPV infection, consider quarterly oral cancer screenings.

Some dentists use supplemental screening devices (Identifi, OralID or Velscope) to shine a bright blue light in your mouth. The light causes pre-cancer and cancer cells to stand out from healthy tissue.

4. Get a biopsy immediately for any suspicious lesion.

If your dentist recommends a biopsy to test cells for cancer or refers you to an ENT or oral surgeon, do not delay! Early diagnosis and treatment can literally save your life.

5. Stop smoking. Stop chewing.

We know it's hard, but it's still easier than losing your teeth, half your face or your life. The chemical s#*t-storm your mouth and airway is exposed to is a cancer threat in itself. Plus smokers face an increased risk of contracting HPV, which can lead to HPV-related cancer. Learn more in Chapter 42, Cigarettes and Chew.

6. Drink moderately.

Apparently HPV doesn't respect any vices—heavy drinkers are also at greater risk of contracting the virus. And regular alcohol exposure considerably increases the smoker's risk of oral cancer. Learn more in Chapter 41, Alcohol.

Chapter 28:

ERECTILE DYSFUNCTION: FLOSS OR BE FLACCID?

In 2012, one of our favorite peer-reviewed readers, *The Journal of Sexual Medicine,* reported on a small Turkish study of men between 30 and 40 years old. Researchers excluded men if they had diabetes, heart disease or high blood pressure, underwent treatment for gum disease within the past year, were taking oral antibiotics or smoked. After that, they had 162 men left: 80 with erectile dysfunction (ED) and 82 without.

Each of the men was examined by a periodontist—a dentist who specializes in gum disease. His analysis? Although 53 percent of those with ED had inflamed gums, less than half that number—just 23 percent—of those without ED showed signs of gum disease.

After adjusting for age and body mass index, the study concluded that men with periodontal disease were 3.3 times more likely to have ED than those without. That doesn't mean periodontitis causes ED, but it's one of the most convincing arguments we've heard for men to take good care of their teeth and gums.

> ## SECRET
>
> Research shows that erectile dysfunction is associated with gum disease. That doesn't mean not flossing will make you flaccid, but we suggest that it's just too risky to skip it.

The connection

So why the connection between gum disease and ED? Let's take a closer look.

At its core, ED is a vascular issue—it's all about blood flow to the penis. ED is affected by any medical condition that causes blood vessels to narrow. That includes atherosclerosis—hardening of the arteries, high blood pressure and high cholesterol.

But what's another way to damage blood vessels? Gum disease. Periodontitis is a chronic, inflammatory disease caused, in part, by a bacterial infection. The gums and tooth-supporting bone structure slowly shrink away, which leads to tooth loss. By the time we see bone changes, periodontitis has already caused systemic inflammation, which sets fire to the lining of the blood vessels.

And that's not all. These dangerous bacteria can also seep into the bloodstream, cruise along for a while and then burrow into the damaged vessel walls to make a new nest and multiply. As this book details, a vast number of studies link gum disease to heart disease, stroke, diabetes and other serious diseases.

An ounce of prevention

Looks like men need some motivation for better oral health, because research published in the *Journal of Periodontology* found women are almost twice as likely as men to receive regular dental check-ups. And the Centers for Disease Control and Prevention estimate that over 64 million Americans have periodontal disease. Of that number, 56 percent are men and 38 percent are women.

Once again, tobacco also plays a role: Smoking is a significant factor in ED. One study showed that men who successfully quit smoking had more penile rigidity and reached maximal arousal five times faster than smokers who relapsed.

" SECRET

Smoking is a significant risk factor for both erectile dysfunction and gum disease. To keep your teeth and your active love life strong, quit smoking. **"**

Quickstart to health

1. Brush thoroughly at the gumline and keep flossing.

Dr. Susan says, "If you'd told me when I graduated from dental school that I'd be offering this advice, I wouldn't have believed you. But now, hear this: If you want to keep your sex life healthy and happy, take good care of your teeth and gums."

2. Work with your dentist to prevent periodontal disease.

Make sure you get a thorough periodontal exam at each preventive visit. And check your risk of periodontal disease using the screening tool in Chapter 4.

3. Quit smoking.

Get help with your tobacco addiction. Erectile dysfunction is just one more negative impact smoking is having on your life.

Chapter 29

CHAPPED LIPS: NOT SO SEXY

SWEET LIPS, cinnamon lips, lips like strawberry wine ...

For 90 percent of the planet, puckering up is an integral part of romance, signaling the possibility of good things to come. But dry, sore, cracked lips do nothing for your love life—and they could mean more serious trouble.

Summer or winter, the more time you spend outdoors, the more likely your lips are to suffer from the combination of sun and wind. The sun, in particular, is a danger: Not only does it burn and chap your lips, but long-term sun exposure, especially on your lower lip, increases your risk of squamous cell carcinoma (SCC).

SCC can be disfiguring and sometimes deadly. The Skin Cancer Foundation reports 700,000 new cases of SCC each year, with 3,900 to 8,800 deaths. You should be particularly concerned if your lower lip border, also known as the vermillion border, has faded so that your lips blend into your facial skin. This increases your risk of developing SCC.

Stress can also play a role in chapped lips. If you're constantly licking or chewing your lips, you may both dehydrate and irritate them. Saliva is great stuff, but it contains powerful enzymes that aid in digestion and can make your lips even more chapped. Simple awareness may be enough to stop the habit; if it's not, you need a plan for stress reduction.

Kids go through lip-licking phases too. Moms and dads often ask Dr. Susan what they can do to help. We know a few things that don't help: Nagging, good-tasting lip balms and cooling balms that contain potentially irritating chemicals. Like any other nervous tic, it may take a while to subside. Consult a physician if your child seems particularly stressed or anxious.

Chapped and irritated lips may ironically result from a contact allergy to the chemicals in the very product we buy to prevent or treat our chapped lips. Scrutinize the labels of the products you or your children use for possible offenders. These include propyl gallate in lipstick, guaiazulene or sodium lauryl sulfate in toothpaste, or red dyes or cinnamon flavoring in everything from candy to mouthwash.

Various medications can also make you more susceptible to chapped lips, so check the side effects for any medication you take on a regular basis.

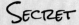

Secret

Chapped lips can be a symptom of many diseases, from diabetes to autoimmune diseases like Kawasaki disease and Sjögren's syndrome. Consult your physician immediately if you notice additional symptoms that cause you to suspect a systemic disease.

The best treatment is prevention

Most people worry more about treating chapped lips than they do about preventing the damage in the first place. The best treatment is to maintain sun protection by repeatedly applying a lip balm with a minimum SPF of 15.

But when you choose your protective balm, take a look at the ingredients first. Dr. Susan sees many patients who have a bad reaction to the lip balm itself, resulting in lined, corrugated, cracked or inflamed lips. Most of those reactions are from cooling agents, which makes it smart to stay away from balms containing menthol, phenol or camphor altogether.

Realize also that by the time you finish a lip balm, you have eaten it entirely. That may make it far more palatable to choose only those filled with natural oils and waxes, such as beeswax, organic olive oil, organic palm oil and evening primrose oil. Avoiding preservatives may mean the balm won't stay fresh in your golf bag until next summer, but it's much healthier for you overall.

If you have any lip ailment that persists for more than a few weeks, visit your physician or dentist to have it examined. They can help determine how serious the problem is and the best way to treat it.

Quickstart to health

1. Don't just treat chapped lips, prevent them.

To protect your lips from the sun and reduce the risk of squamous cell carcinoma, use a lip balm with a minimum SPF of 15.

2. Don't lick or chew your lips.

All the benefits saliva brings to your mouth don't extend to your lips. There it dehydrates the skin and can irritate it also. If you're licking or chewing due to stress, better to work it out with exercise or meditation. If you really need to reduce stress and anxiety, ask a professional for help.

3. Be aware of potential allergens.

Anything that touches your lips could be an allergen that causes them to peel or crack. Frequent irritants include candy, cosmetics, toothpaste and mouthwash. Eliminate suspected allergens one at a time to identify the culprit.

4. Check your medications for side effects.

Many medications may cause lips to dry, chap and crack as a side effect. If you suspect a connection, ask your physician for input and a new prescription.

5. Consult your physician or dentist if chapped lips persist.

If you have chapped lips that last more than a few weeks or don't respond to treatment, see your physician or dentist. This could be a symptom of a more serious illness or condition.

Chapter 30

BAD BREATH: Is It Something I Ate?

NOTHING RUINS A ROMANTIC MOMENT faster than a slow lean-in for a kiss—followed by a fast lean-out for a breath of fresh air. And the heartbreak of halitosis won't just ruin your love life: It's also a faux pas in the workplace, at school or anywhere other people may catch a whiff of breath that could stop a moose in its tracks.

The first question most people ask is this: Is it something I ate? Maybe. You do need to consider the impact of foods on the odors you radiate. Certain foods, including onions and garlic, are absorbed into the bloodstream and expelled from the lungs in the air you exhale. While they may be healthy foods, they can temporarily create breath strong enough to ward off Dracula. Allium expert Eric Block, author of *Garlic and Other Alliums: The Lore and Science,* recommends raw kiwi, eggplant, mushrooms or parsley to tone down the smell.

> ## SECRET
>
> Short-term bad breath is usually caused by something you ate. But long-term bad breath means your oral or overall health is at risk.

The long of it

Bad breath from foods is a short-term problem. But if your bad breath is a 24/7 menace, you may have an oral health problem.

Sometimes the solution to halitosis is simple. If you don't brush and floss daily, for instance, food particles and bacterial growth on your teeth, gums and tongue can cause noxious odors. That's even more of a problem if you wear dentures, but the solution is simple—clean your dentures daily. And be certain to brush your tongue, as well as your teeth or, better still, pick up a tongue scraper.

You may also have periodontal disease with pockets where you've lost bone and your gums have unzipped from your teeth. These pockets harbor more bacteria as well as dying tissue, which can produce the rank odor known as "perio breath." Think rotting flesh. Your dentist can diagnose and treat gum disease, which will not only clean up your bad breath but also decrease your risk of systemic illnesses like heart disease and stroke.

Other common causes of foul breath include tooth decay, yeast infections in the mouth, respiratory infections, chronic sinusitis, post-nasal drip, diabetes and gastrointestinal disturbances. Controlling the secretions in the back of your throat can be challenging; if this is an issue for you, see your physician.

The medications you take may also cause smelly breath. Similar to food, the medication itself may produce an odor after it's absorbed into the bloodstream and exhaled from the lungs. But more seriously, a side effect of many medications is dry mouth, which limits salivary flow. That's bad news, because saliva rinses away some bacteria to clean your breath. Changing medications may improve the air.

If you use tobacco products, whether you inhale or chew, then you have the particularly unpleasant mouth odor known as smoker's breath. As a smoker you're also likely to suffer from gum disease and dry mouth, two significant factors that contribute to bad breath.

Clearing the air

If you go to your grocery or drug store, you'll find shelves of mouthwashes, mints and gums that promise to leave your breath minty fresh. That's true—but they last only a few moments. Then it's back to breath that could make mint wilt.

To find an effective long-term solution that works for you, start with your dentist. He or she will help determine if your bad breath stems from an oral health problem. If not, it's time to see your physician for further investigation.

Quickstart to health

1. Watch what you eat.

We love onions and garlic as much as you do. But if you're planning a rendezvous or asking your boss for a raise, today is not the day to enjoy these potent chemical weapons.

2. Brush at least twice a day and floss once a day.

You need to remove food particles and bacteria that can not only lead to bad breath but to gum disease, which can also putrefy your breath. Be sure to brush the top of your tongue also, where smelly plaque likes to form a coating.

3. Find a solution for your dry mouth.

If you suspect your bad breath is caused by your medication itself or by the dry mouth it causes, discuss alternatives with your physician. Also read Chapter 21, Cotton Mouth.

4. Stop using tobacco products.

Smoker's breath is a noxious odor that's particularly hard to mask—plus tobacco users are more likely to suffer from gum disease and dry mouth, all contributors to knockout breath (and we don't mean that in a good way).

5. Visit your dentist for a personalized solution to bad breath.

Your dentist will determine if an oral health issue causes your bad breath. If so, treating the problem will usually eliminate the smell. If your dentist suspects a systemic problem, he'll refer you to your physician for follow-up.

Chapter 31

MOUTH SORES: SIGNS AND SOLUTIONS

As TEENAGERS, we all had to deal at least once with a zit that blossomed at just the wrong moment and took over our face (or so it seemed at 16). Ultimately it healed three days after the big dance and we did not meet with the social ostracism that seemed certain.

But a mouth sore is a different animal. Whether you're young or not-so-young, you may experience one or more in your mouth or on your lips or face. The unsightliness and discomfort alone may cause you grief. Mouth sores can also be signs of far more serious health problems. Only one type of sore we discuss here directly impacts your sexual health, but which one do you have? Being able to tell them apart could help you avoid becoming infected or spreading disease to others.

> " **SECRET**
>
> There are dozens of oral blisters and ulcers that could mean nothing—or something serious. Check with your dentist if a sore doesn't heal within two weeks. "

Canker sores

A canker sore, a.k.a. aphthous ulcer, occurs on wet tissue: cheeks, gums, soft palate and the underside of your tongue. The sore appears as a rounded, flat, white patch with a red border and can last up to two weeks. If you've had one, you know it's usually painful, especially in high-traffic areas, where the lips or tongue can rub against it.

Researchers still haven't identified the root cause of canker sores, so the bad news is that you can't do much to prevent one. The good news is that they aren't contagious. They're often stimulated by trauma, such as a toothbrush jab, cheek bite or food scrape.

Quickstart to health

1. Treat the pain.

The best remedy Dr. Susan has found is a dab of tincture of benzoin applied with a cotton swab. The benzoin stings for a few seconds and then … Ahhhhhh, relief! Then dab the sore with Orabase B, an ointment that forms a protective coating. Both products are available over the counter, but don't use benzoin if you have an iodine allergy.

Cold sores (aka herpes)

A cold sore usually occurs on the lip or near where it is first contracted from another person. Cold sores are typically caused by the herpes simplex I virus (HSV-1), which is highly contagious.

Repeat this, especially if you're a teenager: *There is no safe sex!* If someone with a cold sore performs oral sex, this can spread HSV-1 to the genitals and cause herpes sores there. In fact, HSV-1 and HSV-2 are equal-opportunity viruses: Either can cause a herpes sore on the face or genitals.

Your first episode will be the worst. A "primary herpes onset" is often accompanied by swollen lymph nodes and/or fever. But soon the sensation morphs into the blister stage. The tiny blisters then rupture into an open sore or multiple sores and eventually scab over—about two weeks from start to finish.

There is an old—and sick—joke that goes like this: "What's the difference between marriage and herpes? Herpes lasts forever!"

That's right: Once you've experienced an episode, the virus is yours forever. It's stored in the ganglion (the techie name for "base") of the nerve and takes advantage of you when you're already down. Another cold sore erupts when your immune resistance is low, like when you have a cold, or experience another insult, such as a sunburn or scrape. The herpes virus creeps out on the same nerve path, so your cold sore usually erupts in the same area each time. There is no known cure, so beware: We can treat only the symptoms.

Quickstart to health

1. Avoid spreading the virus.

Let's repeat this too: Whether it's oral or genital, the herpes simplex virus is highly contagious. From the first tingling sensation, the dreaded sign that a new sore is on its way, you must avoid sharing drinking glasses, straws, forks and smooches or oral sex with another person.

2. Take antiviral medications.

In the past decade, we have shifted treatment to antiviral medications, such as acyclovir (Zovirax) and valacyclovir (Valtrex). Taken as directed, these can help decrease the size of the sore and length of time you have it. These are prescription medications (capsules and ointments) and are most effective when taken orally, from the first tingling.

Angular chelitis (corner sores)

This common mouth sore can wreak havoc with your sex appeal. *Angular chelitis* is an opportunistic infection that makes one or both corners of your mouth look red and puffy. The sore begins with a little crack but, once it gets inflamed, it seems to take forever to heal. We constantly move our mouths, which irritates these sores; but even worse, these cracks breed fungus and bacteria, further challenging the body's ability to heal the wound. The fungus is *Candida,* a yeast, and it loves to grow in dark, moist, warm places, just like these cracked open sores. *Candida* stays especially busy at night, a time when we should be healing.

Angular chelitis can be an even worse problem for denture wearers. If your denture teeth are worn out (or built too short to begin with), your lips become "overclosed." This causes deep corner frown lines that stay wet with saliva and greatly increase your susceptibility to angular chelitis. The dentures themselves can also harbor the fungus and easily reinfect the corners of your mouth.

Quickstart to health

1. Do nothing.

Unfortunately, most people let angular chelitis heal on its own. We don't recommend this as a solution. It's painful, frustrating and takes a long time.

2. Buy over-the-counter remedies.

You can buy topical ointments that can help clear the sores in a few days. Remedies include antifungal ointments containing clotrimazole, antibacterial ointments like Neosporin® and steroids like hydrocortisone.

3. See your dentist.

Prescription versions of the ointments mentioned above are more powerful yet. If you are prone to repeated cycles of angular chelates, your dentist will help you manage the sores. Dr. Susan has had particularly good outcomes with Kenalog in Orabase, a topical steroid ointment that hardens like a second skin. This definitely won't boost your sex appeal, so she recommends you apply it at night as soon as you notice any cracks at the edges of your mouth.

4. Don't touch!

Your hands are covered in bacteria that help feed angular chelitis. So wash your hands often and don't pick at the sores.

Other sores

Sometimes sores are signs of a disease that impacts the entire body. One sign of Crohn's disease, for example, is small mouth ulcers found between the gums and lower lip or along the sides or base of the tongue. Typically the ulcers occur during severe flare-ups of inflammatory bowel disease and back off when it comes under control.

There are dozens of oral blisters and ulcers less common than the three we've covered. If you notice any oral lesion that remains unhealed after two weeks, consult your dentist. It's worth getting a diagnosis. If it's cancer, early diagnosis will save your life.

Quickstart to health

1. Make a dental appointment.

Don't think of your dentist as a tooth doctor, but as the physician who takes care of your entire mouth. Dentists are skilled at identifying mouth sores, just as physicians are skilled at identifying diseases of other parts of your body. Of course, you'll want to let your primary care physician know about any repeated issues with mouth sores.

2. Ask your dentist and physician to work together.

If you experience repeated mouth sores along with other bodily symptoms, it's time for your dentist to work hand-in-hand with your physician. Together they can find the underlying cause and develop a plan to treat you.

Chapter 32

Snoring: The Sexual Buzzkill

RECENTLY MONA CHALABI, lead writer for DataLab, turned to the SurveyMonkey audience for information on the percentage of couples who sleep apart—and why they do it. Almost half of the 1,057 respondents—who were either married, in a domestic partnership, in a civil union or cohabitating with a significant other—said they had slept apart from their partner at least once. Some 14 percent of the couples said they sleep apart every night.

But why do they sleep apart? Mona gave the survey respondents a laundry list of possibilities and the #1 was … (drumroll, please) …

Snoring, checked by 46 percent.

But we're talking about sleep, not sex … right? Right. And wrong. Unlike most animals, who are generally particular about where they sleep but not about where they have sex, humans tend to do both in the same location. Sure it's possible to have a great relationship and separate bedrooms, but that's not what most people want.

Mona asked respondents whether they agreed that "our sex life has improved as a result of sleeping in separate beds." Not so much. Of the 482 respondents, just 5 percent agreed; 40 percent strongly disagreed.

Obviously the impact of snoring on personal relationships can be severe. Nothing ruins your good night's sleep or amorous feelings like your partner, mouth wide open, producing up to 80 decibels—somewhere between the sound of intense traffic and a car horn. Oh you're hot and bothered, but not in a way that promotes good sex! Instead the words "justifiable homicide" may ring in your ears.

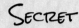

The deafening snore

So what causes snoring? It's simply a sound made in the upper airway as you breathe in during sleep. As your muscles relax, the tongue presses on the flabby tissue at the back of the throat and the airway starts collapsing. Air rushes through this narrowed airway space and the increased turbulence causes the flabby tissue to flap.

And we're not exaggerating when we say it can be deafening. In some cases the decibel level of snoring is louder than what the Occupational Health and Safety Administration (OSHA) allows in the workplace. The din may even cause measurable hearing loss for snorers' bedmates, according to a study published in the *Journal of Otolaryngology.*

According to the American Academy of Dental Sleep Medicine, some 40 percent of adult men, 24 percent of adult women, and 10 to 12 percent of children snore. And as the snorer gets older or gains weight, the snoring gets worse. Time makes tissues in the throat sag and vibrate more; weight gain causes fat deposits to narrow the air passage even more.

Of course, from a dental standpoint, dry mouth (and lack of salivary flow) due to snoring can lead to various oral health problems, including bad breath, infections and sores, tooth decay and gum disease.

But even more critical is the impact on your airway, particularly if snoring develops into obstructive sleep apnea (OSA). We've included further information on this life-threatening disorder in Chapter 19, Obstructive Sleep Apnea.

By working together with your physician, dentist and bed partner, you can find a solution for snoring that improves your overall health and keeps your loved one from wandering down the hall.

Quickstart to health

1. Undergo a sleep study.

If you have obstructive sleep apnea (OSA), you need to know that so you can get appropriate treatment. For snoring and mild OSA, you may need only an oral appliance to keep your airway open.

2. Lose weight.

Being overweight or obese directly impacts the size of the upper airway. The more you weigh, the narrower the airway becomes.

3. Cut down on alcohol and sedatives.

Alcohol and sedatives cause your breathing passages to relax even more, increasing the risk of snoring. Learn more in Chapter 41, Alcohol.

4. Quit smoking.

Tobacco causes inflammation and swelling, which in turn can cause your air passages to narrow. Learn more in Chapter 42, Cigarettes and Chew.

5. Breathe through your nose.

If your nasal passages aren't open, you're more likely to breathe through your mouth. So you can try a few tricks to help keep them from becoming clogged. A steamy shower before bed can help, as can rinsing nasal passages with a salt-water solution. Nasal strips can also be used to lift nasal passages and keep them open.

6. Sleep on your side or stomach.

Sleeping on your back increases the likelihood that the tissues of your mouth and throat will block your air passages.

7. Get surgery.

A surgeon can eliminate the soft palate and uvula—technically known as the hangy-down thing at the back of the mouth. For more severe cases, which include the diagnosis of sleep apnea, it's possible to reposition the upper and lower jawbones to help prevent airway collapse.

SECTION 9

Tooth Function

WE'RE GOING TO START THIS SECTION with a little-known fact even your dentist may never have mentioned. But it can cause you untold pain and suffering.

Here's the naked truth: You can visit your dentist twice a year, brush and floss daily, dodge tooth decay and gum disease, and still experience jaw and facial pain that torments you night and day. That's because the *health* of your teeth and gums also depends on their ability to *function* correctly.

Here's an example. You've probably heard someone say "I have TMJ," which means they have a temporomandibular joint—a jaw joint. What they really mean is that they're experiencing pain or dysfunction related to one or both of their TMJs. Up to 75 percent of us suffer from issues with this joint at some point. And because it's the most complicated joint in the body, treatment can be challenging. Learn more in Chapter 33, TMJ.

Bruxism, which we'll cover in Chapter 34, is another functional disorder, basically a fancy word for teeth grinding. If you think you can skip this chapter because you don't grind your teeth, note this: 95 percent of people do at some point in their lives. You really think you're in the 5 percent? Habitual grinding can wear down your teeth and cause cracks or fractures severe enough to lose teeth or the structure that supports them. But if you know the symptoms and signs of grinding, you can address any issues with your dentist before a costly repair and restore is necessary.

Chapter 33

TMJ:
From Jaw Joint Pain to Chronic Headaches

From the chair

WHEN I MET ANGELA AS A NEW PATIENT, *I was immediately struck by the 32-year-old accountant's impeccable hair and dress. But her dull eyes told the real story. Four or five days a week, Angela suffered from headaches, which she thought might be migraines brought on by work stress.*

I examined her, including a look at her TMJs. Her range of motion was normal, but her right jaw joint was quietly clicking. Several of her chewing muscles were tender to my finger pressure, inside and outside her mouth, especially around her temples and near the jaw joints themselves. I followed up with a thorough TMJ and muscle exam.

Angela went home that day with a mini "bite splint"—also called an "anterior deprogrammer"—to wear at night. I suspected the device would help with her pain, but even I was surprised by the email I received from Angela two weeks later.

"You are SO my hero! I didn't know how distracting my headaches were until now."

I love that kind of email! Almost nothing I do is more gratifying than releasing a patient from chronic pain.

TMJ stands for temporomandibular joint, the ball-in-socket joint where your lower jaw fits into your head, just in front of your ears. (see TMJ diagram on page 7) The TMJs are the most complicated joints in the body, thanks to the ability to hinge both by rotating in the socket and sliding forward. But until one side or the other makes noise or causes pain, you probably never give your TMJs a thought.

SECRET

Human TMJs have tremendous mobility, letting us articulate speech and make facial expressions no other mammal can. We can move our lower jaw up and down, forward and back, and from side to side. The joint movement is so unique that reliable surgery to fix or replace it doesn't exist. To avoid debilitating pain, protect your TMJ function.

How TMJ disorders (TMDs) happen

TMJ noise occurs when the disc—a little piece of cartilage that cushions the ball-in-socket connection—slips partially out of position ... and then slips back. Usually you'll notice a click or pop. You may hear from a TMJ regularly but not feel any pain, so you assume it's normal. It's not. A clicking or popping sound in your joint is still considered a dysfunction.

If your joint or jaws *are* painful, it's usually muscle soreness causing it. The many chewing muscles can become overworked and tender or may even spasm, like a charley horse. This pain often results from clenching or grinding your teeth—and clenching and grinding are triggered by a lack of harmony between your bite and the way your jaw joint *condyles* seat in the *fossas*—or more plainly, the way the balls seat in the sockets.

You can think of the relationship between the jaw joints and the bite as a three-legged stool. When the two TMJ balls are seated solidly in their sockets and the third leg, the bite, is off, you have an imbalance. This TMJ-to-bite imbalance

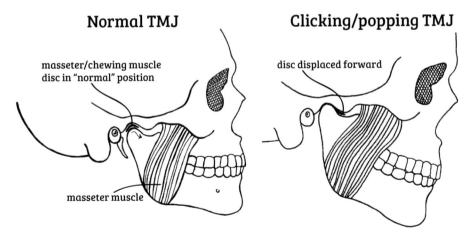

Normal TMJ

masseter/chewing muscle
disc in "normal" position

masseter muscle

Clicking/popping TMJ

disc displaced forward

creates interferences that you may unconsciously try to grind out, often while you sleep at night. That's why many TMJ sufferers complain of morning headaches. But some grinders also work during the day.

The pain may not hover over the TMJ, so it can disguise itself in a number of other ways—as a jaw ache, a tooth problem, an earache, neck soreness or facial pain. More advanced TMD includes locking—a joint that gets stuck open or closed, or a sudden and significant change in your bite, possibly accompanied by a grinding noise. Both of these are signs of the cartilage disc being displaced, squished out in front of the ball.

Sometimes the pain comes from the TMJ itself. If the disc slips out of position for long enough, the result can be arthritis or, even worse, degenerative joint disease. In addition the nerve and blood supply to the jaw joint comes in from the rear of the disc. When the disc slips out of position, these supply lines may be compressed, causing intense pain and inflammation around the ears. The pain can radiate, becoming the source of temple, neck or facial pain and headaches.

> ## Secret
>
> **Disharmony between the proper TMJ position and the way the teeth fit together can stimulate your chewing muscles to work overtime. The muscle spasms that occur as part of TMD can relax when biting harmony is restored, bringing relief from pain and headaches.**

Restoring health

If we were talking about healing knee joint pain, we might prescribe R-I-C-E: Rest, Ice, Compression and Elevation. Unfortunately with the TMJ, we're done before we start, because it's a difficult joint to rest—unless you also give up chewing, biting, speaking, smiling and kissing.

Your TMJ-savvy dentist can help, starting with a thorough TMJ exam and treatment consultation. This exam includes taking a complete history, evaluating range of motion, making load (pressure) tests, measuring the soreness of each of eight pairs of bite muscles and listening with ultrasound to each TMJ.

A proper diagnosis will usually lead to a solution that works to relax your muscles, stabilize your joints and harmonize your bite relationship with your jaw joints. You may need to wear a precision appliance to deprogram your tender muscles.

Most dentists believe in taking a conservative approach to see if simple treatments can improve your TMD. But it's worth persevering to find a solution that works and lets you wake up pain-free every day.

Quickstart to health

1. Visit your dentist.

Your dentist can conduct a thorough TMJ exam and then offer appropriate treatment. If he or she doesn't have advanced training in TMD, you'll probably be referred to a dental specialist who does.

2. Wear a custom-made bite guard.

A bite guard—also called a bite splint, night guard or deprogrammer—can help relax your jaw and reduce the probability of grinding or clenching your teeth at night. Dr. Susan advises against an over-the-counter bite guard. It might protect teeth from the damage of grinding, but it can actually encourage clenching or grinding and wreak havoc with an irritated TMJ.

3. Correct your bite relationship.

This might include slight additive or reductive reshaping of your teeth to create harmony between your bite and your stabilized TMJs. In more serious cases, you may need orthodontics or even "orthognathic" surgery, which aligns the upper and lower jaws, to create a better TMJ-to-bite relationship.

4. Seek physical therapy.

In addition to dental treatment, physical therapy such as ultrasound, heat and ice, and stretching and strengthening exercises can speed muscle healing.

5. See a counselor about stress reduction.

If you think your TMD is exacerbated by stress, counseling may help you find other ways to cope. Lifestyle changes such as regular sleep patterns, frequent exercise and good nutrition are other effective ways to alleviate stress.

6. Review your current medications.

A variety of medications list "bruxism," a.k.a. tooth grinding, as a side effect. If you suspect medications may be contributing to TMJ issues, ask your prescribing physician to consider a different medication.

7. Take medication for TMD.

During the course of your treatment, your dentist may use muscle relaxers, such as Valium or Flexeril, or even strong pain medications on a short-term basis. But don't agree to long-term medication for TMD pain relief.

8. Get injections of Botox to relax muscles.

Some patients get relief after receiving Botox injections to temporarily alleviate chewing muscle spasms. Injections into the TMJ itself are not recommended.

9. Avoid surgery for the TMJ.

Arthroscopic and full-blown TMJ surgeries have been used historically to repair or replace painful joints. Although these surgeries can alleviate immediate symptoms, they often result in more arthritic deterioration. In fact, Dr. Susan, along with the National Institute of Dental and Craniofacial Research, strongly recommends against TMJ surgery.

Chapter 34

BRUXISM: THE NIGHTLY GRIND

From the chair

MY HEALTH RELATIONSHIP COORDINATOR, *Jean, recently estimated that half of our new patients over 40 show wear on their teeth from grinding. That's not surprising: The American Dental Association says about 95 percent of Americans grind or clench their teeth regularly at some point in their lives. That's almost everyone—and the problem is that most of us don't know we're wearing away our teeth unless we wake up with sore jaw muscles, joints or teeth, or tension headaches.*

When I first saw Chuck, a 56-year-old business owner, he had been grinding his teeth for decades—and he didn't know it. Although he visited a dental office regularly, it wasn't until a new dentist took over the practice that Chuck learned flat molars, worn eye teeth, jagged edges on the front teeth, and vertical crack lines aren't normal.

His new dentist explained that Chuck was probably causing the damage by grinding his teeth in his sleep. He offered to make Chuck a night guard to protect him from further wear. But to restore his teeth to their original appearance and function, Chuck needed to see a restorative dentist with advanced training.

When Chuck came to see me for an evaluation, his teeth were worn down to about one-third their original size. His teeth were so short that he needed a gum lift to uncover enough of each tooth to put a lasting crown on. One tooth was abscessed from the wear and could not be restored, so we replaced it with an implant.

One year later, Chuck had a handsome smile and a precision-made bite splint he was committed to wearing at night. But if his grinding had been identified and treated years before, he could have preserved his teeth and avoided a costly restoration.

So many of us grind our teeth that the resulting damage or even loss of tooth structure may be looked at as normal wear. But that's risky if you want to keep all of your teeth for a lifetime. What you lose in tooth structure, you never get back. That's why dentists have a techie name not only for grinding—*bruxism*—but also for the loss of tooth structure from excessive grinding—*occlusal disease*. If you want to avoid spending a hefty sum on repair and restoration, you need to address the problem.

If your dentist doesn't mention grinding, ask if your teeth show signs of it. To diagnose bruxism or occlusal disease, dentists rely on the hard evidence—everything from chipped teeth to greater tooth sensitivity to exposed dentin to jaw or facial pain. We'll tell you more about the clues in the Warning Signs section, so you can talk with your dentist about any indications you might be wearing away your teeth.

Secret

Teeth grinding can result in dramatic loss of tooth structure, which cannot be replaced. But grinding can also be a warning that you suffer from other potentially deadly disorders during sleep, including obstructive sleep apnea and acid reflux.

How bruxism and occlusal disease happen

Tooth grinding has a number of possible root causes. Anxiety, anger and frustration can certainly play a role, but they're not the only triggers for grinding. The body likes harmony, so we tend to grind our teeth when we don't have it.

1. Occlusal or bite interferences: Perhaps the most common cause of tooth grinding is *interference bruxism*, which results from slight interferences in the way the teeth fit together. If your TMJs are in their sockets and any of your teeth get in the way of a smooth closure, it can cause an unconscious irritation—enough to get your muscles busy, working your jaws, to smooth it out.

2. Obstructive sleep apnea: Nighttime airway restrictions can cause stress to the body and trigger bruxism.

3. Drug reactions: Prescription and over-the-counter drugs often list bruxism as a side effect. This includes commonly prescribed drugs like antidepressants, but also overused everyday drugs, like caffeine, tobacco and alcohol. Illicit drugs, including methamphetamine and Ecstasy, are known culprits for severe bruxism.

4. Acid reflux: Stomach acid that shoots up through the throat and airway causes irritation that can stimulate short episodes of waking and swallowing, as well as nighttime grinding.

6. *Neurologic origin:* Most grinders do their work during rapid eye movement sleep, also known as REM sleep. But a small percentage of bruxers grind during the delta wave stage. This *central nervous system (CNS) bruxism* is harder to stop, even with a well-made bite splint. Neurologic diseases such as Huntington's and Parkinson's diseases can also cause grinding.

7. *Age:* Many children grind their teeth at some point or another, especially during the irritation of losing old and gaining new teeth.

8. *Emotional stress:* Stress can aggravate any one of these risk factors. Also, having an aggressive, competitive or high-strung personality type can increase your risk of bruxism.

Warning signs of bruxism and occlusal disease

What clues will tell you that you may be grinding your teeth and damaging your tooth structure?

1. *Chipped or fractured teeth:* Excessive pressure breaks teeth, fillings, crowns and dentures. Even small cracks in your enamel spread like cracks in your car windshield and can result in a fracture when you least expect it.

2. *Sensitive teeth:* If you're a grinder, your teeth may be sore when you wake up or be super-sensitive to cold. That's because bruxism can excite the nerve inside the tooth.

3. *Loose or moving teeth:* Sometimes bruxism can cause teeth to wobble or drift, because the bone around them becomes soft. If this movement isn't controlled, it can result in tooth loss.

4. *Cervical notching or "abfraction":* The flexing pressure of grinding can cause micro-cracks at the neck of the tooth, resulting in a v-shaped notch at the gumline. If the grinding isn't controlled, any filling your dentist puts into that abfraction will break down too.

5. *Sore muscles and facial pain:* Overusing your chewing muscles will make them as sore as the quadriceps of a runner the day after a marathon.

6. *Headaches:* Tension headaches, especially the ones in the temple areas, are most frequently caused by sore, overworked muscles.

7. *TMJ discomfort or dysfunction:* Grinding puts vertical force on the jaw joints. An earache, joint tenderness, restricted range of motion, popping, clicking and/or grinding noises, or locking joints may be a direct result of clenching or grinding. Learn more in Chapter 33, TMJ.

Restoring health

Pay attention to changes in your teeth that might be the result of grinding and discuss the potential causes with your dentist. He will examine any damage with you and perform a TMJ and occlusal exam. He may recommend that at night you wear a precision-made appliance—called a bite splint, bite plane, night guard, anterior deprogrammer or maxillary anterior guided orthotic (MAGO for short)—to help you stop grinding.

If you're tempted to pick up an over-the-counter night guard at your drugstore to protect your teeth, think again. These soft, chewy devices may protect your teeth but actually encourage your grinding habit.

For interference bruxism, *equilibration* can be a helpful treatment. It's a precise bite-adjusting procedure that balances your bite in harmony with stable TMJ positions.

Your dentist can also help you identify lifestyle contributors, such as sleep disturbances, overuse of caffeine, nicotine and alcohol, and prescription or illicit drugs that stimulate grinding as a side effect.

If you suspect the bruxism is exacerbated by stress, take steps to manage it, including better nutrition, daily exercise and therapy.

And if you're showing signs of severe stress, anxiety or anger and have an aggressive or competitive personality, consider tooth grinding an early warning sign that you need to address not just your tooth function but also your overall physical and mental health.

Quickstart to health

1. See your dentist if you suspect signs of tooth grinding.

During a thorough exam, your dentist will see signs of grinding. She'll be able to diagnose the type of bruxism and provide a solution that works for you. If your dentist dismisses the damage you see as "normal" or "nothing to worry about," get another opinion.

2. Consider lifestyle remedies.

Better nutrition, sleep and exercise can help alleviate grinding. Phase out substances that stimulate grinding, including caffeine, nicotine, alcohol and recreational drugs. Address prescription meds with your prescribing physicians.

3. Wear a bite splint at night.

Consider a bite splint that's precisely made to ensure harmony with stable, home-base TMJ positions.

4. Discuss equilibration with your dentist.

Your dentist might also offer a precise bite-balancing procedure to get rid of any interferences that stimulate grinding.

SECTION 10

THE ORAL IMPERATIVE

From the chair

"Of the entire ectoderm—the whole outer covering of the body—what biological structure never repairs itself?"

The question came from a red-haired, freckle-faced fifth grader who wore the biggest pair of Reeboks I'd ever seen on a guy only 4'11".

"Your teeth?" I guessed.

"Right! We learned that in my science class," he said, flashing his own teeth with a smile.

Think about it. If you color your hair pink or shave off the right side, wait eight weeks and you'll get a do-over. The ectoderm includes hair, skin, nails and the cornea of the eye, all of which will heal or grow back if they're injured.

But not your teeth! Every tiny bit of enamel you lose, from decay, wear or injury, is gone forever. So you'd think we'd spend more time and effort caring for our teeth than fixing our hair or doing our makeup. And yet, even the best-groomed of us can be slapdash about a two-minute task like flossing.

Turns out even brushing is at risk: On a radio talk show, Dr. Susan was asked to respond to a recent poll that shows only 44 percent of men and 37 percent of women brush their teeth twice a day.

So in Chapter 35, Your Toothbrush, Chapter 36, Your Toothpaste, and Chapter 37, Your Floss, we review the basics. The sad truth is, many of us don't know the best way to brush or floss or which toothbrush, toothpaste or floss are right for us. Most of us learned to brush from mom, who learned from her mom, who learned from her mom, who came from a generation that didn't brush or floss at all.

Then in Chapter 38, Mouth Rinses, you'll find out the truth about manufacturers' claims. Do their potions really freshen breath, kill germs, prevent cavities, whiten teeth and give them that just-polished feel?

And in Chapter 39 on Fluoride, we'll tell you how dentists first learned that this mineral could prevent decay and also how fluoride's effects differ depending on whether you add it to a water supply or apply it to the tooth surface.

Yes, we're getting back to basics here, but we couldn't leave out this critical section after telling you over and over again to brush and floss. Here's the information you need to take meticulous care of your mouth—and by extension, to contribute to your entire body's well-being.

Chapter 35

Your Toothbrush: A User's Guide

IF YOU WANT TO PROTECT YOUR TEETH AND GUMS from decay and disease, you want the most effective tool out there. But if you go into any grocery or drugstore, you're likely to be mesmerized by shelf upon shelf of choices. Soft, medium and hard brushes, new-fangled or traditional bristle patterns, picks or not, big heads or small, manual or battery-powered, brands old and new, in a rainbow of colors and designs.

Such a smorgasbord of options wasn't always the case. The first bristle toothbrush was invented in 1498 in China. The stiff bristles were taken from the back of a hog's neck and attached to bone or bamboo handles. And that was more or less the only choice for almost five centuries.

Thank Dupont de Nemours for taking pigs out of the picture and introducing nylon bristles in 1938. Their popularity exploded when the army gave toothbrushes and toothpaste to soldiers in World War II and insisted they brush twice a day. Americans influenced by the soldiers' discipline adopted the nylon toothbrush, along with the habit of using it daily.

Which brings us back to what you should look for in your bristly pal's performance. If we made a list of the key criteria, here's what it would look like:

1. First, do no harm. We borrow this from the Hippocratic Oath physicians take. But here we simply want to make sure your toothbrush does not scrub too hard and traumatize your teeth and gums.

2. Clean our teeth and gums. We want a toothbrush that helps us remove food particles and plaque from teeth and gums, and make our mouths feel clean.

3. Look cool! That's where the fun comes in—and why not have a toothbrush that's stylish, shapely, high-tech, sophisticated and/or colorful?

Now let's look at your choices in greater detail.

How hard should it be?

There are hard brushes, medium brushes and the only kind of toothbrush you should consider: the soft bristle brush.

And that's not just because we say so. Soft bristles are the only bristles recommended by the American Dental Association and just about every practicing dentist you'd want to visit.

You don't feel clean unless you give your teeth a hearty scrub with a medium- or hard-bristled brush? We say you like to live dangerously.

Fact is that scrubbing with medium and hard bristles are a major cause of gum recession—from trauma. When the gums recede from the teeth, it's irreversible, except through surgery.

Recession exposes the "cervical" root surfaces—the neck of the tooth, where the enamel ends and the root begins. Root surfaces are covered with a thin and delicate layer of cementum. Cementum is easily scrubbed away, exposing the inner layer of tooth structure, the dentin.

Dentin is seven times softer than enamel—and therefore seven times more susceptible to erosion, abrasion and decay. We call this decay root caries and you can read more about it in Chapter 6, Root Decay. It's a huge issue in this era of sugary, acidic foods and dry mouth from prescription medications.

Exposed dentin is also easily abraded—worn away and notched by scrubbing or by abrasive pastes. Dentin is also more susceptible to erosion from acidic substances, such as lemon-lime drinks. Some root exposure hurts and some doesn't, and sometimes it comes and goes. But patients often ask Dr. Susan about a sensitivity to hot, cold, sweets or even the touch of a toothbrush and learn that the cause is related to root exposure.

A better clean

In addition to a choice of bristle stiffness, manual brushes come in a variety of sizes and styles, but don't be fooled by the package. Can you use the brush easily on the gumline of all your teeth, from the tongue side and the cheek side? Smaller brush heads are often better for hard-to-reach areas. To use a manual toothbrush well for cleaning takes time—but there's an alternative.

Enter the power brush. Studies reported in *Pediatric Dentistry* and the *American Journal of Dentistry* consistently show that no matter what your age, no matter which power brush you choose, it will outpace your manual toothbrush in plaque removal and therefore reduce inflammation.

This is obvious even to a child. Dr. Susan's young patients test this science in the Hands-On Learning Lab™ at her practice. The hygienist smears peanut butter on her gloved hand. The children remove the peanut butter with a manual brush and then with a spin brush to compare the effectiveness. The superiority of power brushes is clearly evident even to a 5-year-old.

And both a 5-year-old and a 95-year old can effectively use a power brush, because the brush does all the work. That's what makes a power brush great for people with arthritis, physical disabilities or other limitations.

But which power brush should you buy? Dr. Susan says rechargeable brushes are more effective for adults than external battery-driven brushes. Spinning brushes, with oscillating and rotating bristles, have different action than sonic, with bristles moving quickly back and forth, but neither seems to consistently outperform the other.

All power brushes tout different features, including quarter or quadrant timers so you know when to move on, and power controllers and interchangeable heads for hard-to-reach areas. In Dr. Susan's experience, most patients who try a power brush immediately notice the more polished, cleaner feel.

Dr. Susan's hygiene team feels the Oral-B® Braun spin brush is the best bang for the buck, although some patients prefer the sonic and more expensive brushes.

Brushing 101

No matter which brush you use, technique matters. In case you haven't had a toothbrushing lesson since you could barely reach the sink, here's a reminder.

1. With any toothbrush, point it toward the gumline at a 45-degree angle. With a manual brush, you'll want to make gentle circles. With a power brush, you just guide the brush along the gumline and let the tip of the bristles do the work.

2. Brush the inner gumline and outer gumline surfaces and also the chewing surfaces on the back molars. Inside the lower front teeth, you might need to position the brush vertically to get bristles on the gumline.

Use of a traditional toothbrush

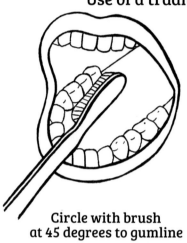

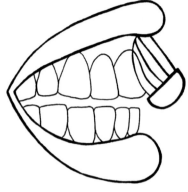

**Circle with brush
at 45 degrees to gumline**

**Keep brush at 45 degrees
to gumline in front**

3. Pay particular attention to brushing inside your lower front teeth and the cheek side of your upper back teeth. These are the areas where the biggest salivary glands empty out—and the saliva can harden up leftover plaque.

> ## Secret
>
> Saliva carries salts that, in just 24 hours, can convert plaque to calculus or tartar. Once the plaque is cemented on, it's there until your hygienist scrapes it with a sharp instrument.

4. Brush your tongue from back to front. Your tongue harbors millions of bacteria, but you can scrape a lot off with a little brushing. This helps lessen bad breath as well.

How long is long enough?

Remember that any plaque you leave behind can start causing trouble by hardening into calculus, aka tartar. And brushing properly takes time.

How much time? A minimum of two minutes. Most people get bored long before that and don't completely remove the plaque.

That's one more reason why power toothbrushes with timers are so valuable. With a beep every 30 seconds, you can divide your mouth into quadrants and spend adequate time on each.

Use of a power toothbrush

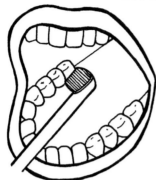 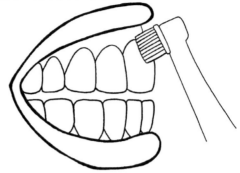

**Guide brush slowly
at 45 degrees to gumline**

**Keep brush at 45 degrees
to gumline in front**

Make a note: We said that doing a good job takes time, not pressure. If your toothbrush starts looking like a scrub brush, frayed out on the edges, you're applying too much pressure. Scrubbers should consider switching to a spin brush, which will help you adopt a new and more effective technique. But if you don't want to change to a different type of toothbrush, try brushing with your other hand. That takes you off auto-pilot mode and forces you to focus on gentler brushing.

So how many times a day do you need to brush? The literature says one thorough cleaning in a 24-hour period will do the job. The problem is we aren't that thorough. So Dr. Susan recommends at least twice a day, but you get extra credit for brushing three times a day.

Any more than that, and you get demerits for brushing away your teeth and gums. Keep in mind that a thorough cleaning includes the surfaces your toothbrush can't reach—so it's better to brush and floss once a day than to brush three times a day and floss once a week.

Quickstart to health

1. Choose a soft-bristled brush.

The American Dental Association and every dentist worth his drill recommend soft-bristled brushes to avoid trauma to the enamel, roots and gums.

2. Make sure you can use the brush to clean all the surfaces of your teeth.

The main purpose of a toothbrush is to clean the surfaces of your teeth from both sides. If the design of your brush or the size of the brush head doesn't allow that, pick another brush.

3. Consider a power brush for more effective plaque and stain removal and reduced inflammation.

The dental literature shows that power brushes consistently outperform manual brushes. In addition, power brushes can be used properly even by individuals with limited dexterity, including young, elderly and disabled brushers.

4. Brush at a 45-degree angle to the gumline.

This angle helps remove bacteria and prevents buildup at and under the gumline. Pay special attention to the inside of your lower teeth.

5. Brush for at least 2 minutes, not including flossing.

That's how long it takes to do a thorough job. If you get bored, picture a toothless crone and see if you can gain inspiration from that.

6. Use a light touch.

Let the tips of the bristles do the work. Scrubbing vigorously can traumatize the gums and cause them to recede.

7. Brush two to three times a day.

Brushing twice a day is the minimum to make sure you're removing bacteria and plaque that contribute to tooth decay and gum disease.

8. Don't store your power brush on an active charger.

Rechargeable batteries are getting better but, like most electronic devices, you'll extend the batteries in power brushes by using them until the power is drained, then recharging them.

9. Replace your toothbrush regularly.

By regularly, we mean every few months to avoid a germ fest. When you get sick and get better, think about pitching your brush to avoid reinfection.

Chapter 36

Your Toothpaste: Finding the Perfect Match

ADVERTISING PIONEER CLAUDE HOPKINS changed Americans' oral hygiene habits forever with a Pepsodent® campaign launched in 1929. The country faced growing oral health issues, but the clever advertisements linked toothpaste to beauty instead—and specifically to getting rid of the nasty film making Americans' teeth dingy.

Hopkins' campaign worked so well that sales exploded and the company couldn't keep up with orders. Pepsodent quickly became an international sensation. If you'd like the whole story, pick up Charles Duhigg's fascinating book *The Power of Habit*.

The advertising has changed, of course, but you'll still find Pepsodent on the shelf of your local grocery or drugstore, along with a wall of other toothpastes that make both beauty and health claims: to protect against cavities or remove plaque and tartar or whiten your teeth or leave your breath fresh or all of the above.

But with so many choices, which one is the best? If you read the ingredient list, you may be more confused, not less. What are all these chemicals? And are they necessary or even healthy for you?

" Secret

If your gums become irritated after using a flavorful new toothpaste, you're probably sensitive to it. Switch to a kids' toothpaste or to the original formula of an old standby like Crest®. "

What's in your toothpaste?

To help guide you, let's demystify the components of various toothpastes:

• **Abrasives** scrape away food particles and plaque. Beware of products not approved by the American Dental Association. Also remember the best de-plaquer is the action of the toothbrush bristle, not the paste.

• **Surfactants** (detergents) and foaming agents clean your teeth by reducing surface tension and creating a slippery film.

• **Fluoride** helps the outer tooth structure—enamel and the cementum/dentin of exposed root surfaces—resist decay. Fluoride also helps make your teeth less sensitive and fights harmful microbes in your mouth. The dental profession considers it the most healthful ingredient to have in your toothpaste.

• **Anti-tartar agents** help to delay the formation of hardened plaque (tartar or calculus). Choose this if you're having trouble controlling tartar buildup despite good brushing and flossing techniques.

• **Desensitizing agents,** other than fluoride, help diminish temperature sensitivity. But it's best to ask your dentist to help you identify the cause of your sensitivity—such as cavities, gum disease or recession, bone loss or tooth grinding—before attempting to treat it with toothpaste.

• **Binding agents** and humectants keep your toothpaste smooth and gooey.

• **Whitening agents** claim to whiten your teeth, but studies show they aren't particularly effective for changing tooth color. They may help with surface stains, however.

• **Sweetening agents** make the toothpaste taste better. They're typically sugar-free additives, such as xylitol, saccharin or sorbitol. If you are sensitive to any of these, be sure to read the label before you buy.

• **Flavoring** masks the taste of all the other ingredients we just listed. Dr. Susan has heard that when manufacturers conduct surveys asking adults how they want their toothpaste to taste, they ask for stronger, more intense flavors. (Remember that a portion of the adult population smokes, which dulls their tasters.) Toothpaste manufacturers keep responding. But the flavor component in adult toothpaste causes gum sensitivity for many patients. If your gums are sore, red, puffy or sloughing, you can try switching to a kids' toothpaste or even Crest original formula. If a toothpaste ingredient is causing your gum inflammation, your sensitivity should subside in about a week.

Which toothpaste should you choose?

With all the choices out there, you can find a toothpaste that specifically meets your needs. Work with your dentist and hygienist to find the best paste for you. But no matter what, we recommend buying one with the American Dental Association seal of approval. At a minimum, it will contain a mild abrasive, fluoride, surfactant, binding agent, humectant and flavoring.

If you are particularly cavity-prone, your dentist may prescribe a paste that packs more power against decay. This includes a higher level of fluoride; xylitol, a sugar that shuts down acid production by cavity-causing bacteria; and calcium hydroxide, a substance that can help remineralize enamel. Dr. Susan's favorite is CTx4 gel by CariFree®.

Quickstart to health

1. Read the label before you buy toothpaste.

If it contains ingredients you don't need—say for sensitivity or tartar buildup—it's not the right toothpaste for you. Buy the toothpaste with the minimum number of ingredients that will work. And if you want whiter teeth, learn more in Chapter 25, Tooth Lightening.

2. Choose toothpaste with fluoride.

Fluoride makes the outer tooth surface more resistant to decay, fights harmful microbes and makes your teeth less sensitive. We like that.

3. Only buy toothpaste with the American Dental Association seal of approval.

The ADA has approved a variety of toothpastes, including regular, sensitive, plaque-prone and organic versions. That means there's one out there that's perfect for you.

Chapter 37

Your Floss: A User's Guide

BACK IN 1999, Dr. Michael F. Roizen, a preventive gerontologist working at the University of Chicago, wrote a book he called *Realage: Are You as Young as You Can Be?* The premise: For better or worse, your biological age may not reflect your chronological age. Roizen created a quiz based on a list of 100 health-related factors. Take the quiz and you could determine your "real age."

Not surprisingly, *Realage* quickly found its way to the New York Times bestseller list. Either we knew we were younger than our birth certificate said and wanted confirmation; or we knew we weren't and needed help. The book contained up-to-date information on all the factors that made up the quiz, from use of tobacco and alcohol, diet, and legal and not-so-legal drug use to marriage satisfaction, parental health and pet ownership.

But particularly interesting were Roizen's comments on oral health. He states that "gum disease is the leading cause of inflammation in the body, which causes aging of the arteries and can lead to impotence, premature wrinkling, heart attack, stroke, diabetes, decreased immune function, and other organ damage." Roizen adds that "flossing daily and regular professional dental cleanings are the equivalent of being 6.4 years younger."

> " **Secret**
>
> Gum disease is among the leading causes of inflammation in the body. Given the links between inflammation and serious systemic diseases, flossing may be one of the best things you do for your overall health—even if you don't live an extra 6.4 years. "

Yes, you need to floss

We're certain that if we could add 6.4 years to the lives of everyone who flosses daily, than the half of people who don't floss would quickly take it up. But adding a health-enhancing habit to your life takes purpose and discipline—you need to be inspired by the positive difference flossing can make and repeat the behavior until it's automatic.

Unfortunately, the majority of people still think brushing is required and flossing is optional. But most of us who are daily flossers can't imagine a day without it.

One of those is comedian, television host, actress, writer and producer Ellen DeGeneres. In her starter ideas for happiness in the book *The Funny Thing is* … she says, "Floss, every day floss … flossing encourages healthy gums and makes your teeth feel secure when they're eating something difficult like apples or corn on the cob."

Flossing cleans the sides of your teeth—the surfaces that you can't reach with the bristles of your toothbrush—and, as Ellen said, is mandatory for the health of your teeth, gums, jawbone … extending right on to your heart and other critical organs.

To reap the full benefit, you need to floss correctly. Correctly doesn't mean you just flick it between your teeth. That's enough to remove a stuck piece of popcorn but not enough to scrape the sticky plaque layer off the sides of your tooth.

Flossing 101

Before we tell you how to floss, you may wonder when to floss: before or after brushing. It matters not, as long as you do a thorough plaque removal at least once a day. Keep in mind that the brush and the floss do the same thing: They both rub off food and bacteria. The brush gets the cheek and tongue sides of each tooth and the floss gets the other two sides. So don't worry about when you floss—just make sure that you do it!

Here are the steps to follow to floss correctly:

1. Start with about 18 inches of floss. Wind most of the floss around one middle finger and the rest around the other. Pinch the floss between your index finger and thumb so you have just an inch or two to work with.

2. Begin with the back surface of the back teeth and move systematically around the arch. That way you can be sure not to miss any surfaces.

3. Ease the floss past the contact and then curve the floss around the side of the tooth in a "C" shape.

4. Wipe the floss up and down gently a few times. The surfaces below the gumline are the most critical, so press as far down as you can, until you meet a natural resistance.

5. Then curve the "C" shape in the opposite direction to clean the next tooth in the same manner.

Use of floss

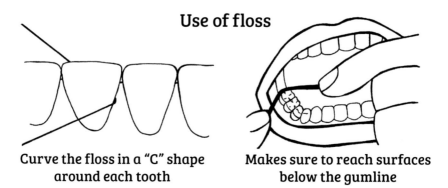

Curve the floss in a "C" shape around each tooth

Makes sure to reach surfaces below the gumline

6. Move to new sections of floss as you go from tooth to tooth by unwinding from one middle finger and winding on the other.

7. Keep going until you're done. In areas where there are periodontal "pockets," where bone loss has occurred, the floss will likely not reach bottom. So how do you access these deeper pockets? Take a look at Floss alternatives below.

Tell your dentist about any area that is a bleeding site or regular food trap, because these areas can lead to permanent bone loss.

The right floss for you

So what type of floss should you use? There are several types, including waxed, unwaxed, woven and tape. All of these do an excellent job of removing plaque and particles as long as you use a careful and thorough technique.

Traditional floss is made by twisting together a number of nylon filaments of various thicknesses and then waxing the floss or not. This type of floss generally works well, but if your fillings or crowns are rough, the floss may fray or tear. In that case, you should alert your hygienist and dentist.

For tight contact points, consider the easier slide of PTFE floss (short for a word so long that we'll just call it Teflon®). It's made of a single filament, so it almost never shreds when you slide it between your teeth. Some of Dr. Susan's patients feel the PTFE floss doesn't remove as much plaque as nylon, however. The truth is, as long as it is interrupting the plaque layer that sticks to the tooth, it's effective.

Floss alternatives

Many patients tell Dr. Susan they're not coordinated enough to floss their teeth, they don't like to put their hands in their mouth or they just can't find the time. But with a multitude of floss aids and alternatives on the market, there's a way for just about everyone to form a flossing habit.

Any widget that suspends a little piece of dental floss can do the same task as traditional floss if used properly. Again, keep in mind that to create the "C" shape, you must put some pressure against the side you are cleaning. Floss aids make it easier for people on the go. In fact, Dr. Susan sometimes suggests her patients store floss aids in their desk drawer or the cup holder of a car. Unlike texting, flossing at a red light is not illegal—yet.

Other aids such as little tapered brushes and tooth picks can also work well. Place one firmly between the teeth, wherever they fit without forcing. If you can insert these aids from the tongue side as well as the cheek side, even better.

Dr. Susan's favorite floss alternative: Stim-U-Dents®. These triangular toothpicks are made of orangewood, so they swell and become more pliable when they absorb saliva. To use them, insert at the gumline, wherever they fit comfortably, broad side toward the gums and pointed side toward the teeth. Push firmly. Toothpicks (even round ones) have the added benefit of compressing the gum tissue and helping disrupt the plaque layer.

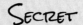

" Secret

Despite claims to the contrary, the best tool for effectively removing attached plaque on the sides of the teeth is floss. That makes flossing one of the best habits you can adopt to protect your overall health. **"**

Water jets

If you already have between-the-teeth pockets—from periodontal disease or bone loss—neither floss nor the alternatives above will be completely effective at cleaning them. Your gums will stop the floss from reaching the lowest dip of the pocket. So what can you do to prevent further bone loss there? And how can you clean other hard-to-reach areas, like under bridges and around braces or implants?

Here's the ideal application for water jets, like those from Waterpik® or Interplak®. These tools send a firm jet of water between teeth and literally create a vacuum that sucks unattached bacteria up and out. Plus any water rinsing helps soften plaque, so it can be more easily rubbed off with other interdental aids.

Water jets work using Bernoulli's principle, which says that as a fluid moves faster, the pressure drops. That's what lets water jets vacuum as well as flush, ringing out food particles and reducing bacterial load.

If you have more acute infection, the water jet can be filled with a prescription antimicrobial rinse that will help you heal better than any antibiotic you take as a pill.

A water jet is also an excellent tool for flushing food and unattached bacteria from hard-to-reach areas, such as under bridges and around braces or implants. And patients with limited dexterity also find it a wonderful aid.

But here's the caveat: Despite the claims that "water jet is clinically proven to be up to 93 percent more effective than flossing," it doesn't take the place of flossing or brushing. Nothing but mechanical scraping can effectively remove this attached plaque. If you don't remove attached plaque every 24 hours, it starts to build hard calculus or tartar. And after that long, the bacteria pool under it gets scarier.

For now, nothing replaces floss. But tools like water jets can provide additional cleaning that make them a great supplement to your oral care routine.

Quickstart to health

1. Floss at least once daily to remove attached plaque.

Flossing is the most effective way to clean plaque from your teeth and keep your teeth, gums and bones healthy.

2. Make sure you use good flossing technique.

Good technique requires forming a "C" shape with the floss around every tooth and rubbing it up and down.

3. Choose the type of floss that you prefer.

The best type of floss is the type you'll use at least once a day. If that's nylon or Teflon, woven, waxed or unwaxed, cherry or mint, we approve.

4. Use a floss alternative if you can't floss well or if you floss more often with a tool.

If your flossing skills are lacking, choose a tool that makes flossing easier for you. That could be anything from a floss holder to a toothpick.

5. Ask your dental hygienist for tips on flossing.

Your hygienist will be happy to watch and coach you on the correct way to floss to keep your mouth healthy.

6. Add a water jet to rinse away unattached plaque.

Water jets can suck unattached bacteria from your mouth to reduce the bacterial load and the inflammation it can cause. Patients with deep gum pockets, bridges, braces, implants, or limited mobility find it's a wonderful aid to clean thoroughly.

7. Tell your dentist and dental hygienist about any area that's a bleeding site or regular food trap.

These can be signs of gum disease, leading to permanent bone and tooth loss and increasing your risk of a heart attack or stroke. Your dentist and dental hygienist can help you make sure your gums stay healthy and your teeth stay in them.

Chapter 38

Mouth Rinses: Swishing Off the Claims

YOU BOUGHT A MOUTHWASH that claimed to freshen breath, kill germs, prevent cavities, whiten teeth and give them that just-polished feel. Sounds like a dream come true, doesn't it? Well, like most dreams, some of it is grounded in reality and the rest is fantasy. But which part is which? With so many different mouthwashes on the market, it's hard for you to know which one is best—or even if you need a mouthwash at all.

Before we look at the claims mouthwash manufacturers make, let's start by considering the environment where we want it to work. You can picture tooth enamel as a bundle of tiny glass straws or tubes. The ends of the straws at the tooth surface suck up liquid in the surrounding environment. At the same time, the mucosa—the wet skin of the gums and tissues—are also part of this environment.

Secret

Rinsing the mouth, even with plain water, causes the plaque on your teeth, gums and tongue to absorb the liquid and swell. That makes it easier to remove the plaque with a toothbrush and floss.

Be wary of claims that a rinse can take the place of using your trusty brush and floss for scraping off plaque. Any mouthwash needs to be an add-on to your normal oral hygiene routine, not a substitution.

Claim #1: Freshens breath

Let's face it, many people buy a mouthwash to cover bad breath. While the intense odor neutralizers in mouthwash do work, the result is usually short-lived. The typical mouthwash on your grocery or drugstore shelf cannot address the underlying cause of continual bad breath.

For persistent odor problems, consult your dentist to look for signs of gum disease (rotting flesh smell), cavities (rotting tooth smell), food impaction (rotting food smell), smoking-related gum disease (rotting rotten smell) or other oral infections.

Claim #2: Kills germs

Some mouth rinses have "antimicrobial" bacteria-killing additives that reduce gingivitis or plaque—or so they say. Listerine has been the most popular over-the-counter antimicrobial rinse and is somewhat effective at ridding your mouth of microorganisms.

The problem is that the antiseptic essential oils must be dissolved in alcohol (27 percent ethanol) to work—and alcohol rinses are not recommended for long-term use. Some studies reveal that swishing alcohol against the mucosa on a habitual basis can increase the risk of oral cancer. In addition, mouth rinses with alcohol can dry out your mouth, making it harder for saliva to do its job of cleaning plaque and debris. Johnson & Johnson responsibly reformulated a less effective but alcohol-free product called Listerine Zero®. The point: Just say "NO!" to any mouth rinses that contain alcohol.

Chlorhexidine ups the effectiveness. Not only does it have an antiseptic-sounding name, but it is also considered the most therapeutic antimicrobial substance you can put in a rinse. In fact, chlorhexidine is added to most doggie toothpastes on the market to help reduce gum infection and tooth loss. Your pooch can get it over the counter, but you'll need a prescription.

The most common for-people prescribed products containing chlorhexidine are Peridex® and Periguard®. These are prescribed for short-term home care, but dentists and hygienists squirt chlorhexidine into deep pockets to help less active gum disease.

Claim #3: Prevents cavities

So what about using a mouthwash for cavity protection? Fluoride is the not-so-secret ingredient you're looking for. Fluoride molecules clog up the glass straws in your teeth that we told you about earlier. Clogging sounds undesirable, but actually it helps protect the tooth from absorbing dangerous acids in the vicinity.

The problem here is that over-the-counter rinses don't contain an effective concentration of fluoride. The Food and Drug Administration regulates how much fluoride can be put in a single bottle, in case the bottle is accidentally swallowed. For example, the concentration in a large bottle of ACT® is actually less than in the smaller bottle, because the company is held to a maximum allowable amount per bottle.

Still, some fluoride is better than no fluoride, so if you're hooked on mouthwash, look for one with fluoride.

But if you're truly looking for a solution to a cavity problem, ask your dentist for a prescription rinse that contains a more "efficacious" fluoride concentration. For her cavity-prone patients, Dr. Susan likes the CTx series by CariFree. The rinse has a powerful fluoride component, but instead of a minty flavor it has a mild bleach taste. That's due to the inclusion of sodium hypochlorite, which neutralizes acids in your mouth to further guard against decay.

Claim #4: Whitens teeth

You'll find many mouth rinses that claim to whiten, lighten and brighten teeth and none that do it well. Those glass straws require enough time to suck up the lightening agent and influence the inner layer of tooth structure known as the dentin. You'd have to hold a rinse in your mouth a very long time and, even then, the results wouldn't make you smile.

Claim #5: Gives your teeth that just-polished feel

Be skeptical of rinses that make your teeth feel smooth too. Detergents or surfactants reduce the surface tension of the liquid it's in, which creates a slippery film over everything in your mouth. Your tongue will say "oooooh, ahhhhh," and your plaque will thank you too for *not* removing it.

In short, no mouthwash can substitute for good oral hygiene, regular preventive dental exams and professional cleaning. Your best bet may be to rinse with water before brushing and flossing rather than using any of the "cosmetic" mouthwashes. If you have specific problems for which you need a solution, let your dentist prescribe the right short-term therapeutic mouth rinse for your situation.

Quickstart to health

1. Rinse with water before you brush and floss.

Plain water will loosen plaque and food debris as well as any other liquid, including the best-marketed mouth rinse. Swishing with water makes it easier for your brush and floss to do their job.

2. Nix mouthwashes with alcohol.

Alcohol is used to preserve the active ingredients in antibacterial mouthwashes. But studies have linked regular swishing with alcohol-concentrated mouthwashes to oral cancer. In addition, alcohol can dry out your mouth to the detriment of your oral health.

3. Consider a mouthwash with fluoride.

Fluoride can help prevent cavities by protecting against acids in the mouth. But over-the-counter mouth rinses generally don't contain enough fluoride to do a lot of good. Your dentist can prescribe mouthwashes that are more effective.

4. Save your money on rinses that "whiten."

For lasting results, lightening agents need to be in contact with your teeth for extended periods of time. Your mouthwash will never be in your mouth that long.

5. Be suspicious of mouthwashes that make your teeth feel smooth.

If your teeth feel slippery smooth, it's because the mouthwash contains a detergent or surfactant that coats plaque and debris—they're still there underneath the slick.

6. Consult your dentist about therapeutic rinses for your situation.

For specific oral health issues—persistent mouth odor that can't be tamed, infected and inflamed gums, regular occurrence of cavities or dingy teeth—your dentist can prescribe a therapeutic mouth rinse that will work a whole lot better than anything you can buy over the counter.

Chapter 39

Topical Fluoride Treatment: Is It Worth It?

Dentist Frederick McKay spent 30 years tracking down the natural ingredient that made the teeth of early 20th century residents of Colorado Springs, Colorado, so resistant to decay. You already know the answer—fluoride. Although the controversy drags on over adding fluoride to public water supplies, your dentist may have a simple message about fluoride: It works.

As a cavity-buster, topical fluoride application is arguably the greatest value of the cleaning appointment. Fluoride inhibits decay, desensitizes teeth and slows down the metabolism of bacteria that cause cavities. Repeated exposure to it usually means fewer cavities and fillings.

Dr. Susan's child patients learn about topical fluoride and its effectiveness in the practice's Children's Hands-On Learning Lab™. The kids place a fluoride-soaked egg and a plain egg into a beaker of acid—in this case, white vinegar. The natural eggshell bubbles up, fizzes and even begins to spin. The fluoride-soaked egg sits, inert like a rock, completely protected.

Let's take a closer look at the rationale for fluoride, as well as the pros and cons of the different fluoride delivery systems.

Systemic fluoride

Dentists have historically believed that systemic fluoride—fluoride added in public water systems—was more beneficial than topical fluoride used on the surface of teeth. But the dental literature keeps flip-flopping on which is best. With the increased acidity in our food supply, topical application seems to be winning. But dentists and medical scientists still tout the benefits of systemic fluoride.

Systemic fluoride builds cavity protection into developing enamel before a child's teeth ever erupt through the gums. This creates an inherently stronger, more cavity-resistant structure than enamel without fluoride. The result: a 40- to 60-percent lifetime protection from decay, according to a study in the *Journal of Public Health Dentistry*.

Although many developed countries do not add fluoride to their water supplies, 70 percent of water systems in the United States do. These systems add fluoride salt, also known as sodium fluoride, to drinking water in concentrations less than 1 part per million. The Environmental Protection Agency regulates the amount in accordance with the Safe Drinking Water Act. At such low dosages, fluoride strengthens teeth without proven potential for negative health effects.

The controversy over fluoride revolves around the fact that fluoride used in this way becomes a drug, according to the Food & Drug Administration. And not all the people receiving the treatment necessarily agree to it. But pediatricians and dentists agree that we don't want to miss the window of opportunity to strengthen kids' teeth for a lifetime.

In fact, if you live in a rural area and drink well water, as Diana does, you may want to help your kids' developing teeth with a systemic fluoride supplement. But it's critical to have the water analyzed first, because fluoride can occur naturally and already be present. (Remember Colorado Springs?) Too much fluoride can cause "fluorosis," which results in permanent yellow or brown spots on the teeth. They're strong, protected and really unattractive.

Most county health departments offer water analysis at no or low cost. Take the sample from your kitchen sink where most of your cooking and drinking water comes from. Then share the results with your dentist, who will determine if your children need a fluoride supplement—and the precise amount.

For kids without fluoridated water, Dr. Susan prescribes fluoride supplements, either drops or tablets, based on each child's age and weight. On average she prescribes about 0.1 milligram a day for kids who have no fluoride in water at home or school and half of that for those with fluoridated drinking water at school. Due to the risk of fluorosis, she recommends a professionally calculated prescription.

Topical fluoride

Topical fluoride has grown in importance for children and adults alike—mostly because our diets have become much more acidic than our ancestors' diets. Think of all the juices, sports drinks, sodas and diet sodas we consume, then realize that all of these have a pH (a measure of acidity) thousands of times of that for plain water.

So how do we get topical fluoride? Tap water is one source, albeit a weak one. Toothpastes and over-the-counter rinses are another. But far more effective sources are professionally applied foams, gels, rinses and varnishes, applied to clean enamel surfaces every three to six months.

Dr. Susan's choice is a fluoride varnish applied every six months. Varnishes dry quickly and will set even in the presence of saliva, so there's less gagging and swallowing than with a three-minute tray filled with gel or foam. You also don't need to polish teeth for them to absorb the varnish. The tooth's natural biofilm layer helps the fluoride varnish stay put and absorb into the tooth surface for several hours. And finally, research has shown that fluoride varnishes reduce the number of the cavity-causing bacteria *Streptococcus mutans* by more than 10-fold.

Cavity-prone kids and adults can increase topical exposure with a home fluoride product. Your best bet: Talk with your dentist to develop a fluoride protection plan personalized for you.

Quickstart to health

1. Find out if your water supply includes added fluoride.

Not all U.S. water systems add fluoride. Contact your public or community water company to find out if your children are getting fluoride by ingesting tap water.

2. If you're not on a municipal system, get water tested for fluoride.

If your water comes from a well or private system, get your water tested to determine if it contains the recommended dosage of fluoride to prevent tooth decay—currently 0.7 parts fluoride per million parts water.

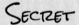

3. Consider fluoride supplements for your children.

If you want to protect your children's teeth with systemic fluoride and your system does not have an adequate concentration, talk with your dentist about calculating the correct dosage for supplements.

4. Get professional topical fluoride treatments.

Professional fluoride varnish is the best choice for topical protection of the teeth already in the mouth.

5. Use fluoride toothpaste and perhaps a rinse.

Daily use of a fluoride toothpaste and mouth rinse can continually replenish the fluoride in the tooth enamel, protecting against decay. These over-the-counter products aren't as effective as formulas professionals can subscribe.

6. Talk with your dentist about a personalized fluoride protection plan.

A custom fluoride protection plan will take into account your systemic fluoride consumption and the optimal topical fluoride treatments to protect your family's teeth from decay.

SECTION 11

Addicted Nation

ONE OF THE BIGGEST CHALLENGES WE FACE as Americans is addiction. But we're not talking about speed, meth, crack, junk or Acapulco Gold here. We're talking about addictions to substances that are perfectly legal and socially acceptable—from prescription medications to sugar, alcohol, tobacco, caffeine and junk food. Our behaviors around these substances are undermining our oral and overall health and upending our healthcare system.

First up in Chapter 40 are Prescription Drugs. That's a major concern to dentists, who often prescribe pain meds after procedures and then confront patients claiming high levels of discomfort weeks afterward. If that seems like a minor issue, be aware that unintentional fatal overdoses involving prescription painkillers now outnumber deaths due to cocaine and heroin combined.

We also drink alcohol to excess, despite all the warnings about moderation. Everyone is aware of negative impacts on the liver, but too few are aware of the increased risk for seven types of cancer, cardiovascular disease and pregnancy complications—to say nothing of tooth decay from the sugars alcohol contains. Learn more in Chapter 41, Alcohol.

Despite all the warnings, some 18 percent of American adults still smoke tobacco and 3 percent still chew. Nicotine remains one of the most addictive substances on the planet. And though far fewer people smoke now than 50 years ago, rates of lung cancer have declined only slightly in the past three decades. Chapter 42, Cigarettes and Chew, will tell you why. And although smokeless tobacco doesn't cause lung cancer, it more than makes up for that by the increased risk for oral cancer.

We also have a national sweet tooth—an average of 128 pounds of sugar a year for each of us. Studies show sugar lights up the pleasure centers of the brain just like cocaine. And it's not the sweet stuff you're adding from the sugar bowl that's the major factor. In the meantime, we're experiencing a worldwide obesity epidemic and rising rates of tooth decay, as we explain in Chapter 43, Sugar.

Sugar also taints sodas, fruit juice, sports drinks, coffees and energy drinks. Yet millions spend most of their waking hours sipping on a combination of sugar and acid that boosts fat stores and rots teeth. Our consumption of sodas has dropped—so why hasn't that solved the problem? Learn more in Chapter 44, The Unholy Trio.

We've added sugar-laded caffeinated beverages to the mix as well. Some 90 percent of Americans consume caffeine, many to beat sleep deprivation. Now 73 percent of kids drink it every day too. The news on caffeine isn't all negative—but we tell you why moderation is in order in Chapter 45, Coffee and Energy Drinks.

Finally, our diet has transformed in the last few generations into one our great-grandparents would hardly recognize. Too many of us rely on flour-sugar-salt-chemical-laden foods for too large a part of our diets. We give you some food for thought—literally—in Chapter 46, Processed Food.

Chapter 40

PRESCRIPTION DRUGS: PAINFUL ADDICTION

IN A NATION WHERE MANY CONDONE "taking a pill for whatever ails you," it's no surprise that prescription drug abuse has become a serious public health concern. According to the 2010 National Survey on Drug Use and Health, an estimated 2.4 million Americans used prescription drugs for recreational purposes for the first time within the past year. About one-third of those individuals were just 12 to 17 years old.

The most common drugs abused fall into three categories: opioids (narcotics) to treat pain; depressants for anxiety and sleep disorders; and stimulants to manage attention deficit hyperactivity disorder.

From the standpoint of your local dental practice, the most serious concern is abuse of pain medications. And from Dr. Susan's perspective, the post-operative painkillers prescribed to teenagers following wisdom teeth removal may play a large role in first-time abuses.

From the chair

Tommy was one of my teenage patients, a high school senior who had his wisdom teeth extracted. His oral surgeon prescribed 28 tablets of Vicodin, which contains acetaminophen and hydrocodone, an opioid that resembles codeine. To me, the original prescription seemed excessive—but then Tommy went back to the surgeon complaining of continued discomfort. The surgeon doubled the prescription.

How did I find out? Certainly not from Tommy. I heard about it from Tommy's tattling little brother during Tommy's dental exam. Even a 13-year-old knew needing that much painkiller was shady.

So I did what any responsible adult would have done; I asked Tommy about it directly.

"Did you really have a lot of pain after the first week? Tell me about that," I said.

"Well, not really," Tommy replied. "But the drugs helped me relax around my friends and I found out they liked my personality better when I was taking it."

The problem is evident. Although painkillers are definitely effective at killing pain, many people really like the slowed, loose feeling of being "high" on opioids—and this triggers drug-seeking behavior and habitual use.

In 2013, of the 43,982 drug overdose deaths in the United States, more than half (51.8 percent) were related to pharmaceuticals—and 71.3 percent of those involved painkillers. Overdoses of prescription pain meds ultimately killed 16,235 individuals.

SECRET

There's a misperception that prescription drugs are less harmful than street drugs. In fact, unintentional overdose deaths involving opioid pain relievers have quadrupled since 1999. By 2007, these deaths outnumbered those involving heroin and cocaine combined.

The unknowing dental dealer

Dental offices often become the targets of drug seekers. In fact, many patients will ask for a prescription even after a very minor procedure. And sometimes a people-pleaser dentist has a hard time turning down a paying customer. Some polished drug seekers already know which dentists are the easy marks. They will talk about pain and even be willing to undergo drastic procedures, such as an extraction that results in permanent tooth loss, to get the one thing they came in for—a drug they can't live without.

Sometimes drug seekers are easy to spot. They may be overly anxious, fidgety and impatient, and dramatic about their symptoms. Others are more difficult to identify, tipping their hand at the end of the appointment with a strong recommendation about exactly which drug and dosage they should be given.

For example, Dr. Susan saw a patient named Michelle for a couple of extractions recently. After five injections of a strong local anesthetic, Michelle's mouth was still not numb.

So the dental team scheduled a new appointment for Michelle on the next day. Dr. Susan tried a different anesthetic and, although Michelle was not profoundly numb, she did get some relief. Michelle asked Dr. Susan to go ahead and pull the tooth, which was painful for everyone involved. When the visit ended, Michelle asked for a specific prescription—a strong narcotic. She proceeded to name, with authority, all the lower forms of narcotic and non-narcotic pain relievers that "just don't work" on her.

Why was it so challenging to numb Michelle's mouth? Digging further, we learned that she has a history of chronic pain and has been taking prescription pain meds a long time. In her case, all evidence indicates that habitual drug use, especially of narcotics, has led to a hyper-tolerance of the anesthetic, making it difficult for her to get numb without high doses.

Is this the fault of Michelle or of all the prescribing docs who preceded this dental visit? Dr. Susan says both play a role. According to Dr. Harold Crossley, an expert on the pharmacology of drugs used in the dental office, prescribers make some common mistakes. Dentists often write prescriptions that aren't necessary and prescribe too many pills even when the prescription is necessary. Often a narcotic-free, over-the-counter, non-steroidal anti-inflammatory drug (NSAID) like ibuprofen is powerful and effective enough to handle the pain from a typical extraction. In fact, Dr. Crossley recommends prescribing whatever dose a patient would safely take for a headache.

Already hooked

Addiction isn't always the patient's fault, of course. Physicians often prescribe narcotics for pain management following major surgery. They are most effective if taken even *before* the pain sets in—in other words, before numbing or sedation wears off. As healing progresses and the pain slowly subsides, the patient should taper the drug. But narcotics are physically addicting, so lowering the dosage can bring more anxiety and discomfort than even the original pain. Some patients report that they must have pain meds just to function, and stopping cold turkey brings on symptoms like sweats, stomach cramps and overall weakness.

If you or someone you love has experienced this scenario, it's best to seek professional help to escape the vicious cycle of detox and relapse that is so common among those who suffer from narcotic addiction. Ask your physician to intervene. Often patients addicted to painkillers need a combination of replacement dugs, counseling and a 12-step program like Narcotics Anonymous to fully recover.

Quickstart to health

1. For dental pain, consider NSAIDs.

Non-narcotic drugs, such as ibuprofen or naproxen, are powerful pain relievers for oral pain. They don't affect the brain, so they are not mood-altering or addicting.

2. Use prescribed opioid pain medication respectfully.

As soon as your pain subsides, taper your intake or transition to non-narcotic meds.

3. Monitor your children's use of narcotic medications.

If an opioid is prescribed for your child following an extraction appointment, keep an open dialogue about pain levels. Don't let your child control how often and how much pain medication he takes.

4. Don't drive under the influence of pain meds.

Even if you think you're feeling fine, your reaction time is slowed from narcotics. If you were in an auto accident, you would be liable for causing it.

5. If you or a loved one is addicted to pain meds, get help.

Narcotic addiction is a serious health threat that often results in permanent organ damage or overdose.

Chapter 41

ALCOHOL: SOBERING TRUTHS

THE AUTHORS OF THIS BOOK have a confession to make: We drink alcohol, mostly wine, but with enchiladas a margarita and, at the ballpark, a beer.

Seems we're in good company. Alcohol is the favorite mood-altering drug in the United States—some 44 percent of us over the age of 18 have downed at least 12 drinks in the preceding year. The main effects of alcohol, both sublimely pleasant and downright crappy, are known widely. The devil is in the details.

We're all aware of the immediate buzz of alcohol, even with just one drink. Despite the images of happy imbibers, alcohol is a depressant. That means it lowers breathing and heart rate, slows reaction time, impairs coordination and vision, and challenges thinking and good decision-making.

Of course, alcohol also causes many long-term impacts, including increased risk of seven types of cancer—not just liver cancer—plus cardiovascular disease and pregnancy complications. And alcohol consumption also increases the risk of oral cancer and the likelihood of periodontal disease, tooth decay and mouth sores that may be pre-cancerous.

Even those of us who drink in moderation are at greater risk for all of alcohol's ill effects, but they're of particular concern for addicted drinkers or those who abuse alcohol by binge drinking. Some 14 million Americans—more than 7 percent of the population—meet these criteria.

> ## SECRET
>
> Individuals who drink alcohol, even at levels recommended for moderation, have a greater risk of oral and pharyngeal cancers. For optimal oral and overall health, consider moderation (two drinks a day for a man and one for a woman) the upper limit of consumption, not a goal.

Journey of a drink

What happens when you down that cocktail, beer or glass of wine? Well, as the saying goes, "Over the lips, past the gums, look out stomach, here it comes!"

Of course, it's not quite that simple. Alcohol hits the lips, tongue, gums and wet skin of the mouth on its way to the upper throat (pharynx), food pipe (esophagus) and voice box (larynx). And yes, it irritates everything it touches, which is why alcohol increases the risk of cancers in these locations. How exactly that happens is not known, but it's thought that alcohol may damage cell DNA.

Ultimately your drink arrives at the stomach, where it also irritates the stomach lining. About 20 percent of the alcohol is absorbed right there in your stomach, while the rest gets taken up by the small intestine. How quickly the alcohol is absorbed depends on how strong your drink is—from beer, at the low end, to hard liquors like vodka, at the high end. Carbonated beverages also find their way into the bloodstream faster. A full stomach slows down the rate of absorption, which is a convincing reason for always eating or at least snacking before you drink.

Once absorbed, the alcohol enters your bloodstream and makes a floating tour of your body until it's removed. One of the stops along the way is the brain, where it slows down all the key functions noted above.

Your kidneys and lungs remove about 10 percent of the alcohol in your urine and breath, respectively. That's what allows a Breathalyzer to effectively measure your blood alcohol concentration.

And finally, the liver bears the brunt of the work, breaking down the rest of the alcohol to acetic acid.

Alcohol and your overall health

Oddly enough, people who drink often think about the damage they could do to their liver or stomach lining, and ignore its impact on other parts of their body. It's true alcohol is the primary cause of liver cancer, as well as liver cirrhosis and trauma. But in addition to the cancers already mentioned, it's also a risk factor for breast cancer and bowel cancer. And it may also play a key role in the development of stomach ulcers.

While we're talking about cancer, let's not forget that those who drink alcohol have a six-time greater risk of oral and pharyngeal cancers. The risk increases with the amount consumed and with binge drinking. By a binge, we're talking about five or more standard drinks for a male or four for a female. Binging is a strong trend among college and high school students.

According to the American Cancer Society, about 70 percent of oral cancer patients consume alcohol frequently. Add tobacco smoking to heavy alcohol consumption and you more than double the trouble, because the two act synergistically. The Oral Cancer Foundation reports that individuals who smoke and drink have a 15 times greater risk of developing oral cancer than those who don't. In fact, the combination of smoking and drinking is the primary risk factory for approximately 75 percent of mouth cancers in the United States. (Persistent human papillomavirus infection is the #1 risk factor for cancers that occur back by the tonsils and throat.)

Is the news all bad for the impacts of alcohol? Almost. You've no doubt heard that the antioxidants in red wine can actually improve your cardiovascular health. But drinking wine is definitely not like eating kale and berries, where more is better. And in truth, maintaining a healthy weight, eating a nutritious diet and exercising regularly will do far more for your cardiovascular health than a daily drink will ever do.

Alcohol and your oral health

Even if you don't have an alcohol dependency, drinking can still undermine your oral health. The issue: Alcohol, even beer, contains sugar—and by feeding the acid-producing cavity bacteria, alcohol can destroy your teeth just like soda does.

Add acidic mixers like soda to hard liquor, and you've got a double whammy. You're a little better off—but not much—with fruit juices and ciders. Wines are also quite acidic and sweet wines give you an extra dose of "residual" sugar.

Alcohol also dries out your mouth, as anyone who's ever experienced cotton mouth can confirm. That means that the saliva that protects your teeth from decay can't do its job. Now we've got a triple whammy.

If you're addicted to alcohol, you deal with all these negatives and more. Alcoholics can be lax about eating a nutritious diet or taking care of their personal hygiene, both risk factors for oral health problems. A study published in *U.S. Dentistry Today* showed that 80 percent of alcohol abusers have moderate to severe gum disease and decayed teeth. More than one-third have potentially precancerous lesions. Alcohol abusers also exhibit poor compliance with regimens to improve and maintain their oral health and poor healing after dental surgery.

Everything in moderation

You've heard the adage before, but in this case moderation lets you enjoy alcohol responsibly. That's critical for both your oral health and your overall health.

So what do we mean by moderation?

Well, men have the advantage here. Moderate drinking means consuming no more than two drinks per day if you're a man and one drink per day if you're a woman.

And yes, we'll define a drink too. A drink means 12 ounces of beer, 5 ounces of wine or 1½ ounces of hard liquor. If you have any question about how much—or little—these volumes are, measure them out yourself.

Even if you do drink in moderation, we encourage you not to drink and drive. Always plan on a designated driver or an alternate way home, such as a taxi or bus. You protect your own health and that of everyone around you, a definite win-win.

And if you suspect you are addicted to alcohol, get help. Alcoholics Anonymous is a powerful and wonderful organization and there are meetings in almost every community in our country.

Quickstart to health

1. Drink in moderation.

That's two drinks for a man, one drink for a woman, with one drink equal to 12 ounces of beer, 5 ounces of wine or 1½ ounces of hard liquor.

2. Seek help if you abuse alcohol or are a problem drinker.

Your oral and overall health, and perhaps your life, are at stake. Consult your physician or go to www.aa.org to find an Alcoholics Anonymous meeting near you.

3. Check with your physician before mixing alcohol with any drug.

If you're taking medications, even over-the-counter drugs, ask your physician or pharmacist about the impact of mixing them with alcohol. The result could be anything from making your medication ineffective to making you severely ill.

4. Before drinking alcohol, brush and floss.

You need to remove the bacteria that would otherwise eat the sugar and spit out acid. It's always a good idea to keep your teeth clean—just be certain not to brush within an hour of drinking acidic beverages, when your enamel is more susceptible to abrasion because of the acid.

5. Drink water and swish it in your mouth when you drink.

Water helps rinse away the sugars and acid from alcohol. In addition, alcohol dries your mouth and dehydrates your cells, so drinking water encourages cell hydration.

Chapter 42

CIGARETTES AND CHEW: YOUR MOUTH ON NICOTINE

HE PASSED ON JUST A FEW DAYS after his 73rd birthday. So he didn't quite make it to the average life expectancy for men of 75. But worse, he spent the last seven years with mounting disability, suffering from one stroke after another.

If he hadn't smoked he might have seen all seven of his grandchildren graduate from high school or even college. Or get married. He might have experienced the joy of adding great-grandchildren to the large family gatherings.

He might have had more Thanksgivings and Christmases and birthdays with his two children and two stepchildren or had more golden years with his wife of decades.

Instead they all remember him for his sense of humor, his playfulness and his generosity. They remember even now how he always had the right answer to any question, because his moral compass was spot on.

It's been more than a decade, but his daughter, Dr. Susan, knows he'd probably still be alive today if he hadn't smoked. After all, most non-smokers live into their eighties. Instead he died far too soon of stroke-related complications.

And to make this more tragic, Dr. Susan remembers the day, just a few years ago, that she realized her dad's advanced, smoking-influenced gum disease posed perhaps a bigger risk factor for his recurring strokes than his smoking. In fact, after the first stroke he quit smoking.

But every year since his death, Dr. Susan re-ups a very personal goal for her dental team in her father's honor: To help at least 30 people quit smoking.

> ## SECRET
>
> Cigarettes today deliver their dopamine reward faster, addict you more readily and kill you more efficiently. In the mouth, they wage a war that results in gum infection, tooth loss and the risk for oral and pharyngeal cancer. These effects serve as a potent warning of the havoc they wreak throughout the rest of the body.

Cigarettes

You're probably well aware of the hazard of smoking cigarettes on your overall health. The danger comes from inhaling chemical compounds, some in the tobacco leaves themselves, some in the 4,000+ chemicals added to protect the leaves in their growing season.

What you may not know is that over the years, cigarettes have become more addictive—and more deadly. Cigarette manufacturers are adding chemicals to today's cigarettes that cause the nicotine to reach the brain much more quickly. Faster delivery of nicotine means faster release of dopamine—the feel-good reward for smoking. Adding menthol has also taken away some of the harshness of smoke, the better to initiate children and teens into smoking.

But cigarettes have become much more deadly as well. According to the *50th Anniversary Surgeon General's Report on Smoking and Health,* lung cancer risk for smokers rose dramatically between 1959 and 2010. The risk for people who never smoked stayed about the same. That's true even though smokers in the 21st century smoke fewer cigarettes a day than earlier smokers.

A century ago, cigarettes were much simpler—no filters, no vent holes, fewer added chemicals. It's thought that these additions may be leading smokers to inhale more deeply, pulling bad stuff deeper into their lungs.

In short, smoking makes you much more likely to die an early death—and suffer for years—from a long list of diseases: lung and other cancers, respiratory diseases including chronic obstructive pulmonary disease (COPD), heart disease, stroke and type 2 diabetes, macular degeneration, autoimmune disorders and compromised immune systems. Women are more likely to experience pregnancy complications and to bear children with birth defects.

Chew

Many people, mostly men under 30, think they'll outsmart nicotine by using smokeless tobacco. They assume these will be less addictive and less harmful than cigarettes. And why not? They see that "dipping" is part of the team culture for great American athletes playing baseball and football. What they don't realize is that nicotine, in any form, gets a firm grasp on you and refuses to shake loose.

Smokeless tobacco comes in two main forms. First there's chew, which is available as loose leaves, plugs or twists. And then there's snuff, a more finely cut or powdered tobacco available loose, in strips or in small pouches that look like tea bags. Whichever you use, it's frosted with those same 4,000+ chemicals in the herbicide/pesticide cocktail. In addition, manufacturers add chemicals to enhance flavor and absorption.

To use either form of smokeless tobacco, you just tuck a pinch between your gums and cheek or lower lip. Your body absorbs nicotine through the mucosa—the cheek tissue—stimulating nicotine addiction and a cascade of other health threats, including cancer.

According to the American Cancer Society, the most common of these deadly life-threatening cancers are oral cancers of the floor of the mouth, tongue, cheeks, gums and throat, not to mention cancers of the esophagus, pancreas and stomach. In addition, smokeless tobacco increases the risk of dying from heart disease and stroke, according to a report in *Circulation*, the journal of the American Heart Association.

Your mouth on nicotine

Closet smokers and chewers may think their secret is safe—but the mouth is a dead (pardon the pun) giveaway. Chances are, your dentist knows if you use any type of tobacco.

Your compromised oral health shows up in a variety of ways:

• Increased risk for gum recession and disease, including gingivitis and periodontitis

• Two times the risk of tooth loss

• *Leukoplakia,* which are white, pre-cancerous changes on the gums, cheek, tongue or floor of the mouth or tongue

• Oral and pharyngeal cancers

• Slower recovery from tooth extraction or surgery

• Excessive buildup of plaque or tartar on teeth

• Tooth decay

• Stained teeth

• Fungal infections, such as thrush or hairy tongue, which looks just like it sounds but comes in colors ranging from yellow and green to brown and black

Dr. Susan is particularly concerned about oral cancer, which shows up as a small, strange spot ranging in color from normal to white, red or black. Often it hides or is disguised by white, ruffled tissue (leukoplakia) present at the site of nicotine absorption in smokeless tobacco users. Oral cancers are hard to detect, especially in that sea of abnormal-looking tissue—and when dentists find them, they're usually seeing a very small part of the underlying cancer.

In fact, Dr. Susan has been shocked when a tiny spot of cancer seen in the mouth resulted in radical removal of parts of the tongue, lip or jawbone, severely disfiguring patients' faces and their quality of life. Despite all the progress we've made in curing other types of cancer, oral/pharyngeal cancer has only a 57-percent five-year survival rate. That means almost half who get oral cancer die within the first five years. For the survivors, the necessary surgical treatments sometimes alter appearance and function so drastically that some patients prefer death.

A quitter always wins

Mark Twain once said, "Quitting smoking is easy. I've done it a thousand times."

Leave it to Twain to get at the truth by poking fun. For those of us who care deeply for someone who battles nicotine addiction—perhaps yourself?—it's a sad truth that nicotine users depend on their drug.

So cutting the chain that drags the ball is not as easy as mind over matter. The nicotine receptors in the brain can stay hungry for "a fix" long after you stop using tobacco. But many people have successfully quit, and you or your loved one can too.

Here are a few tips on quitting strategies:

Quitting "cold turkey" has a miserable 5 percent one-year quit rate (OYQR).

Nicotine replacement therapies, such as the patch, inhalant, electronic cigarettes, gum and lozenges, have an average 15 percent OYQR. Getting your fix through the skin or mucosa is still safer than getting it through the airway and lungs. Although it's easier to switch to another delivery mechanism than to quit nicotine entirely, it doesn't end the drug addiction. Over time, however, folks tend to revert to their favorite form of delivery rather than kicking the habit. But with discipline you can slowly cut your dosage. If you choose to go with gum, try to find a sugar-free product.

E-cigarettes are becoming more popular, because they let users inhale nicotine in a vapor without the damaging tar of conventional cigarettes. Research into the dangers of e-cigs is ongoing, and the FDA is poised to begin regulating the products. A good rule of thumb to remember is this: The only thing that really belongs in your lungs is air.

Zyban/Wellbutrin is a non-nicotine solution that has a 30 percent OYQR. Wellbutrin was originally prescribed as an antidepressant, but physicians in a study club noticed that some patients quit smoking. For the first time in the history of the U.S. Food and Drug Administration, a drug was relabeled for a different purpose. Zyban uses the same dosage and administration—but although Wellbutrin is typically covered by insurance, Zyban is not. As though smoking cessation isn't a serious health problem! Not so incidentally, this drug is associated with weight loss of 11 pounds a year when taken for depression, a counterbalance to the average 8-pound weight gain wanna-be-ex-smokers can anticipate.

Chantix, another non-nicotine solution, has shown a 14 percent OYQR (although the pharmaceutical company claims higher). The most common side effect is nausea, which passes in a week or so.

Hypnosis works with variable results, depending on the therapist and how "hypnotizable" the subject is. Hypnosis is non-invasive therapy—substance-free—which is a bonus.

Acupuncture works amazingly well in the hands of some therapists and is non-invasive as well. In Dr. Susan's community, one acupuncturist for tobacco cessation claimed an 85 percent quit rate in a program paid for by a local community college.

Is quitting easy? No. Can it be done successfully? Yes. Diana's father smoked for 50 years, then lived the last 15 years of his life without one cigarette. How'd he do it? He broke his leg—and by the time he was done with the hospital and rehab, he hadn't smoked in so long he never started again.

As Dr. Susan says "Keep on quitting ... until you get there."

Quickstart to health

1. If you don't use tobacco, don't start.

Nicotine is highly addictive. If you don't start using nicotine, you never have the challenge of weaning yourself away from it.

2. Whether you smoke or chew, quit.

Talk with your health professional, your family and friends or a local anti-smoking organization to plan a quit attempt right for you. The American Cancer Society provides resources to help you quit in their *Guide to Quitting Smoking*, available online. The National Institute of Dental and Craniofacial Research offers an excellent guide for quitting smokeless tobacco called *Smokeless Tobacco: A Guide For Quitting*, available online.

3. Re-think nicotine replacements.

Beware of products that switch one method of nicotine delivery for another. Pay particular attention to the mounting evidence of potential harm from e-cigarettes.

4. Recognize that the cigarettes manufactured today are more addictive and deadly than ever.

Manufacturers have increased the speed at which nicotine reaches the receptors in your brain. In addition, the lung cancer rates for smokers have increased in recent decades, while they've stayed stable for non-smokers.

5. Don't think that smokeless tobacco is healthier.

Yes, you may skip some of the respiratory implications of smoking. But you won't miss out on the chance for a particularly nasty and deadly form of cancer, tooth loss or chronic oral health issues, such as persistent fungal infections.

6. Help a loved one quit tobacco use.

The American Cancer Society provides a list of Do's and Don'ts to help friends and family support someone they love who wants to break their addiction to nicotine.

7. Be extra vigilant about oral hygiene until you quit.

Smokers are more susceptible to oral diseases, including bacterial infections. Visit your dentist more often, get more cleanings, get more exams and be diligent about brushing and flossing.

Chapter 43

Sugar: Anything But Sweet

FIFTY YEARS AGO, around the same time that Neil Armstrong took the first stroll on the moon, the government proposed another lofty goal—to end tooth decay forever. The deadline? The end of the 1970s. Hindsight being what it is, you know we still haven't achieved success. But as a recently discovered archive of documents called the "Sugar Papers" shows, the National Caries Program (NCP) was doomed from the start.

Why? Well, like today, scientists knew that sugar causes tooth decay—a fact accepted since at least 1950, even by a sugar industry trade organization. What the industry didn't accept was any strategy for caries reduction that called for U.S. citizens to eat less sugar.

The industry's stand might not have mattered if the task force that set research priorities for the NCP wasn't littered with physicians and scientists tied to the sugar industry. An analysis of the "Sugar Papers" conducted by Christin Kearns, D.D.S., M.B.A., who discovered the archive, along with Drs. Stanton Glantz and Laura A. Schmidt, showed that in the late 1960s and early 1970s, the sugar industry cultivated relationships with the National Institute of Dental Research (NIDR). The relationships were so close that a sugar industry expert panel included the same individuals—except for one—on an NIDR panel that influenced priorities for the tooth decay program.

You won't be surprised to learn that a full 78 percent of the sugar trade organization's research priorities were directly incorporated into the 1971 NCP's first request for research proposals. Not surprisingly, the request didn't include any research that might harm the sugar industry.

Today the sugar industry's position on tooth decay remains the same—that public health should focus on fluoride toothpaste, dental sealants and other ways to reduce the harm of sugar, rather than reducing sugar itself.

Even given the knowledge that excess sugar is now also linked with heart disease, diabetes and liver disease, the industry opposes current policy proposals, like the World Health Organization's (WHO) newly released sugar guidelines. And the industry remains adamantly against the proposed change to the Food &

Drug Administration's nutrition facts label that would include "added sugar." The change would let you know how much of the sugar in the food you're eating was added during processing.

Dr. Glantz, who was the original recipient of the "Cigarette Papers" that triggered the multimillion-dollar lawsuits against the tobacco industry in the 1990s, sees striking parallels with the sugar industry's strategy: "Our findings are a wake-up call for government officials charged with protecting the public health, as well as public health advocates, to understand that the sugar industry, like the tobacco industry, seeks to protect profits over public health."

> ## SECRET
>
> The public health policies related to sugar consumption could have been addressed 50 years ago. Instead sugar consumption has skyrocketed—and it remains up to you to monitor your intake and keep it within recommended guidelines.

The secret ingredient

You won't be surprised to learn that Americans haven't cut back on sugar consumption—in fact, the U.S. Department of Agriculture (USDA) says the per capita consumption of caloric sweeteners, mainly white sugar and corn sugars, increased 39 percent between the 1950s and 2000. By 2013 the USDA estimated the average American's yearly sugar consumption at 128.3 pounds per person for all 316.5 million of us. With numbers like these, you don't need a panel of experts or the WHO to tell you that the United States has a sugar problem.

Imagine 25 five-pound bags of sugar lined up on the kitchen counter and someone finishing one off every two weeks.

"That's not me," you probably say. "There's no way I would ever do that."

The problem is you may do that and not even know it. Our processed, packaged foods are full of sugar—but because the word sugar seldom appears as one of the ingredients, it's easy for us to live in denial.

We shouldn't be surprised that candies, baked goods, jams and jellies are full of sugar. And you know sweetened beverages contain sugar, although the amount might shock you. You'll also find most breakfast cereals, along with fruit snacks, granola bars, crackers and even salad dressings, chock full of sugar. But why do ketchup, mustard, teriyaki sauce, peanut butter and nut toppings need sugar?

Why? Because sugar is a game changer. The food industry knows that if they add sugar, we will consume more. Not just because the taste is irresistible, but because it influences our body chemistry to want more. Your fat cells decrease the output of the satisfaction hormone called leptin, and your stomach produces a hunger hormone called grehlin—the one that makes it growl. The combination of these drives you to eat, eat and eat some more.

Secret

Sugar goes by 60+ aliases. By one name or another, sugar is tucked into 90 percent of all processed foods. Limiting sugar will help you avoid obesity and type 2 diabetes, which WHO calls epidemics, and tooth decay, which is on the rise.

Packing on pounds

Compared with 20 years ago, Americans are consuming an average of 130 to 260 more calories a day—at the low end for adult women and the high end for teenage boys. If you do the math on unburned calories stored as fat, that's the equivalent of 14 to 28 more pounds per person—per year. You can learn how those extra pounds undermine your health in Chapter 14, Diabetes, and Chapter 16, Obesity.

But where are the extra calories coming from? Mostly from sugar and white flour, which acts something like sugar when you consume it. The obesity trends make sense if you do a little math: If you eat 100 extra sugar calories each day, you gain a pound of body fat every 35 days (every 3,500 calories). In a year, you'd gain 10 pounds—and the fat stored would take up the volume of about two footballs.

Although you may think that your body treats every calorie the same, that's not the case. If you slug down 500 calories of Mountain Dew in the morning to jumpstart your day, you get a sugar rush, then an immediate insulin spike as the body works to clear away all that sugar. Most of the calories will be stored as fat. But an hour later, after your blood sugar drops, you'll be hungry again.

If instead you eat 500 calories of broccoli, you'll be totally stuffed. Your blood sugar won't rise, because all that fiber moves through the gut at a glacial pace. Your insulin won't spike and your body won't get a message to store the fuel as fat. And after 16 cups of broccoli, you won't be hungry for a while.

High-fructose corn syrup and low-fat diets

One sugar source of particular concern is high-fructose corn syrup (HFCS), also called corn sugar, which entered the market in the 1970s and has become a mainstay of food manufacturers. They love it because, as a liquid, it's easier to work with than sugar; it's sweeter than the white stuff; and it's cheap, thanks to the U.S. Government's subsidies to corn growers.

HFCS and table sugar contain roughly equal amounts of glucose and fructose. But unlike glucose that can be used for fuel by any cell, only the liver can break down fructose. One of the end products of that breakdown is "triglycerides," a form of liver fat. The result of chronic overconsumption of fructose? Non-alcoholic fatty liver disease.

So why are we over-consuming sugar and, in particular, fructose? One of the major triggers was the low-fat diet craze that began in the 1970s. Food manufacturers started offering processed foods with a lot less fat—even fats that were healthy for us. But take out fat and often you take out flavor and the mouth-feel that gives us satisfaction. So the manufacturers added sugar or HFCS, plus a bunch of chemicals to help mimic the feel of fat. Check out low-fat peanut butter on your grocer's shelf: It has far more sugar than the regular-fat version.

But given what the liver does with fructose—turning it into triglycerides—we actually kept the high-fat content. In fact, low-fat diets may have been the single biggest contributor to obesity growth, according to Dr. Robert Lustig, author of *Fat Chance: Beating the Odds Against Sugar, Processed Food, Obesity and Disease*. Chronic fructose exposure also leads to insulin resistance—in which the body produces insulin but the cells don't recognize it, so the pancreas keep on pumping—a precursor to diabetes.

One other item worth noting is the research into how regular sugar and HFCS impact the body differently. In a Princeton University study, rats with access to HFCS gained significantly more weight than those with access to table sugar, even when the calories they consumed overall were equal. We should add that the rats were drinking HFCS at rat-sized levels well below those you'd find in your typical can of soda.

In a study reported in March 2015, University of Utah biologists fed mice sugar in doses proportional to what many people eat. They found the fructose-glucose mixture in HFCS more toxic than sucrose or table sugar, reducing both the reproduction and lifespan of female mice. Female mice on the fructose-glucose diet had death rates 1.87 times higher than females on the sucrose diet. They also produced 26.4 percent fewer offspring.

Sugar guidelines

Oddly enough, the FDA has specific guidelines on the amount of salt and fat we eat, but not on the amount of sugar. So we have to turn to the American Heart Association or WHO.

The AHA suggests an upper limit for women should be 100 calories per day, about 6 teaspoons, and for men should be 150 calories per day, about 9 teaspoons.

In its 2014 guidelines, WHO recommended that we lower our sugar consumption by a whopping 75 percent, down to 5 percent of our daily calories. How much is 5 percent? If you are an adult and consume 2000 calories a day—about average for an active person who weighs 150 pounds—5 percent would be about 100 calories. That's 25 grams of sugar, a little more than five teaspoons a day. If you drink soda, just one 8-ounce can already contains more than your daily allotment of sugar.

What about kids? Given children's lower body weight and energy requirements, one 8-ounce soda represents about 10 percent of their total calorie intake, twice what's recommended.

The WHO report is a reaction to the growing epidemics of obesity and type 2 diabetes, as well as the continued rise in tooth decay. Studies confirm decay rates increase in proportion to consumption of sugar in children: "Because dental caries are the result of lifelong exposure to the dietary risk factor (i.e., sugars), even small reductions in risk of dental caries in childhood is of significance in later life," says the WHO document. To learn more about how caries occur, read Chapter 5, Tooth Decay.

WHO also called out the massive consumption of sugar-sweetened drinks in all industrialized countries, such as sodas, sports drinks, energy drinks, sweet tea and juice. (See Chapter 44, The Unholy Trio, for more information.) Not only is the fiber-less, concentrated liquid sugar harmful to the liver, pancreas and tooth structure, but it's also lacking in nutrients that the body needs to ward off inflammation and boost the immune system. And as we noted, it contributes to the triple whammy of obesity, type 2 diabetes and caries.

For the sake of your teeth, your body and your family's health, read labels and control your sugar intake.

Quickstart to health

1. Limit the amount of sugar you consume.

WHO and AHA have both issued guidelines for the amount of sugar you eat. WHO recommends no more than 5 percent of daily calories from sugar; AHA suggests an upper limit of 100 and 150 calories a day in sugar for women and men, respectively.

2. Cut out sweetened beverages.

Concentrated liquid sugar without fiber will give you a glucose spike, followed by an insulin spike. We suggest you eat whole fruit instead of drinking juice, soda, sports or energy drinks.

3. Read labels.

First concentrate on limiting your total sugar consumption, no matter what kind it is. Learn the 60+ names for hidden sugar in processed food and then read the labels on the foods you buy. Make a point of avoiding foods that contain high fructose corn syrup or corn sugar. Remember, if a chemical name ends with —ose, chances are it's added sugar.

4. Recognize that low-fat does not mean low-calorie.

When food manufacturers cut the amount of fat in processed food, they often add sugar to improve the flavor and chemical thickeners to simulate the mouth-feel of fat. You may end up with a product that's actually higher in calories, more fattening and more toxic than its normal counterpart.

5. Put the sugar bowl back on the table.

If you must add sugar to breakfast cereal or fruit, you'd be better off buying the unsweetened variety and adding it directly. You'll never add as much sugar as manufacturers pack into most pre-processed breakfast cereal or canned fruit packed in syrup. And if you can cut back on added sugar, one day you may appreciate the sweetness of a simple piece of fruit.

Chapter 44

THE UNHOLY TRIO: SODA, JUICE, SPORTS DRINKS

A FEW YEARS AGO, Dr. Susan spent a bleak January day examining 17 college students—kids who had grown up in her care, now home for winter break. At the end of the day she felt like crying. All but one of these young patients had new cavities. Instead of shedding tears, she realized she needed an effective way to issue a warning: Sweet drinks are literally destroying your teeth—and adding extra pounds you hate.

For millennia, our ancestors have been savoring the rare sweetness given up by the fructose in fruit and honey. And for centuries we've been savoring the sweetness of sucrose from sugar cane or sugar beets. But our current sugar consumption is unparalleled in human history.

> ## SECRET
>
> Drinks touted as healthy, including 100 percent fruit juice and electrolyte-filled sports drinks, are some of the worst offenders in terms of excess sugar content. The solution: Drink water, steer clear of soda, and guzzle sports drinks only during long or intense workouts.

The sweet life

According to Michael Moss, author of *Salt, Sugar, Fat*, we consume 71 pounds of added sweeteners every year—that's 22 teaspoons of sugar per person, per day. Moss says the amount is split almost equally in three piles: sugar derived from sugar cane, sugar beets and the corn sweeteners that include high-fructose corn syrup (HFCS).

HFCS is the newish entry into the sugar market, a sugar engineered in the 1950s and available for food manufacturers beginning in the 1970s. Since then it has become one of the most successful ingredients ever to hit the market. According to ConsumerReports.org, consumption of HFCS jumped more than 1,000 percent between 1970 and 1990.

And why not? It offered the food industry a low-cost, high-volume solution to sweetening foods. As a syrup, HFCS does not need to be dissolved to be used in applications like sodas. It's chemically stable in our diet of increasingly acidic foods and beverages—everything from baked goods to juice. And it's made of corn, a hardy, inexpensive crop that will still be standing when all else is gone, if we believe the 2014 sci-fi flick *Interstellar*.

Moss reports that since 1970, Americans consumption of sugar-sweetened soda doubled to an average of 40 gallons a year per person—about two 8-ounce cans every day. We're not drinking soda and neither are you, right? So someone out there is getting way more than their share.

Although soda consumption dropped to 32 gallons a year per person by 2011, there's no basis for a *Hurrah!* We've more than made up for it: A spike in the consumption of sweet drinks like teas, sports drinks, vitamin water and energy drinks has filled in the gap, up to 14 gallons a person per year. Add them up and we're averaging 46 gallons a year now … *per person.*

The bitter news

We've mentioned the word "sugar" in conjunction with "decay" often enough in this book that you know where we come down on sugar or HFCS. Given the level of tooth decay among U.S. children and teenagers, we recommend *zero* consumption of sweetened beverages.

From the chair

To illustrate the amount of sugar in your soda or sports drink, take a funnel and a clear, empty bottle of the beverage. Spoon the amount of sugar indicated on the label. For example, if you have a 20-ounce bottle of Gatorade® Lemon-Lime Thirst Quencher in your hand, the top two ingredients are water and sugar. How much sugar? Thirty-four grams per 20-ounce serving. Always check the serving size—otherwise you might mistakenly assume the number of grams represents the whole container. For sugar, 4 grams equals a teaspoon. So this sports ade contains 8.5 teaspoons of sugar. If you sip on it during a typical one-hour workout, it will keep the bacteria in your mouth ecstatic for that time plus an additional 40 minutes or so. Unless your workout is intense, the sugar will cause your insulin to spike and the excess sugar to be stored as fat, which is probably not what you were hoping for from your workout.

With sugar and decay, it's the *frequency* of consumption that poses the gravest danger. By sipping on something sweet throughout the day, you keep the "cavity bugs" fed and they keep kicking out acid. Plus the drink itself is an acid bath.

After you're finished with your beverage, it still takes the saliva up to an hour to neutralize the acidity. If you sip all day, the acid is never neutralized.

One more warning: If you eat or drink something sweet within an hour of bedtime, you create another recipe for disaster. Saliva flow more or less stops at night so, if you nod off when the acid level is high, your teeth will suffer all night long.

Then what about just gulping down your sweetened beverage? Well, if you drink a gallon of a sugared beverage every day, all within 10 minutes, you probably won't get cavities from it. You may suffer from obesity, diabetes, heart disease, kidney stones and other unpalatable diseases, but not cavities.

But better still, reserve sweetened drinks as a once-in-a-while treat. If you must have one every day, drink a modest serving with a meal and be done with it.

The switch

So what can you do? Switch to diet drinks? Yes. The one we recommend is called water and it's free if you get it from your tap. Other diet drinks may eliminate the sugar problem but the ingredient list is scary.

Diet sodas are no longer considered a healthy choice. In a 10-year study of 2,500 over-40 adults, drinking diet pop was linked to a 43 percent rise in cardiovascular disease, including stroke, heart attack and death. Diet sodas are high in sodium too, so it's no wonder they are associated with high blood pressure. But ironically, drinking diet soda was also associated with high blood sugar, diabetes and expanding waistlines.

Dr. Susan is both a dentist and a mom, so she's definitely concerned about the *habitual* (not occasional) ingestion of high-tech chemicals like those in diet sodas.

As a toddler, her son Hunter had the "one finger rule" for all the groceries in their cart: If he couldn't cover the ingredients with the width of his little finger, it wasn't going in the cart. When he started to read, he would pick up a bag of junk food or drink and grimace, perplexed by all the strange words that spilled out under his finger, none of which sounded like food. Now a healthy and athletic 21, he continues to read the labels—not for the calorie count but for the quality of the ingredients.

What about juicing? It's a current trend that certainly sounds healthy. But you're much better off eating the whole fruit or vegetable. Why? The answer is fiber. If you extract the juice and pitch the fiber, you will miss out on the micronutrients in the plant that slow digestion, sugar release and insulin response, lessen fat storage and lower your risk for type 2 diabetes.

A paper published recently in the *British Medical Journal* shows that individuals who consumed at least two servings each week of whole fruits, especially blueberries, grapes and apples, lowered their risk of type 2 diabetes by up to 23 percent. But those who drank one or more servings of fruit juice every day increased their risk by almost as much—21 percent.

Sports drinks are a little tougher, because they supply hydration, sugar and replacement of sodium, potassium and salts. That's what makes them so useful for a long or intense workout. But sports drinks have deviated a lot from the original Gatorade, created for the Florida Gators. Their reformulation has created increasingly sweeter versions and they're consumed mostly by teens who are typically not playing hours of football in the grueling Florida sun.

According to the American College of Sports Medicine, if you're working out for less than an hour, you don't need a sports drink unless you're sweating profusely. That's most likely true even for 90 minutes of exercise in cool conditions.

Longer than that, and you'll need to replace electrolytes and fuel up, as well as hydrate. In that case, sports drinks can prevent overhydration and hypernatremia, a potentially life-threatening condition in which the concentration of sodium in the blood drops dangerously low.

Diana drinks Gatorade regularly when her running workouts last more than an hour. But if she's not working out and just plain old thirsty, she doesn't reach for a sports drink and neither should you. That's when clear, cool H_2O is the perfect drink.

Quickstart to health

1. Be aware of the sugars in all the drinks you consume.

It's easy to think that if sugared soda is bad for you, switching to juice or vitamin water will be a healthy alternative. Not so: These drinks also contain high amounts of sugar. Even those that contain low amounts of sugar will feed cavity-causing bacteria and may result in tooth decay.

2. Drink water to rehydrate.

Water should be your go-to beverage when you're thirsty.

3. Steer clear of diet sodas.

Diet sodas are associated with high blood pressure, weight gain and increased risk of heart attack, stroke and diabetes.

4. Eat fruit instead of drinking juice.

The process for making most juice keeps the sugar and acid intact but destroys the beneficial nutrients and antioxidants, and removes the natural fiber.

5. Consume sports drinks only during long, intense workouts.

Workouts shorter than 60 minutes probably don't require sports drinks, unless you're sweating profusely.

Chapter 45

COFFEE AND ENERGY DRINKS: WAKE-UP CALL

WHEN DR. SUSAN reported to one of her young patients that Mountain Dew® was creating a breakfast drink, he chimed in: "Really? I thought Mountain Dew WAS a breakfast drink!"

Maybe we don't all down Mountain Dew, but 83 percent of adults in the United States drink coffee, according to the National Coffee Association's 2013 online survey. And 73 percent of teens and younger children drink caffeinated beverages daily, in sodas, energy drinks and coffees, according to a study reported in the journal *Pediatrics.*

What is caffeine? It's a white alkaloid powder derived from coffee beans or tea leaves and sprinkled into any liquid. And therein lies the problem. Although caffeine in limited amounts can claim some mild health benefits, it's seldom downed in hot water alone.

Instead it shows up in drinks like a Starbucks caramel latte, Pepsi®, Red Bull® and Rockstar®, where the primary ingredient is not caffeine, but sugar. And as we know, sugar underlies our epidemics of tooth decay, obesity and type 2 diabetes.

From an oral health standpoint, many caffeinated drinks, including coffee, can stain your teeth—but that's superficial and can be scraped off. For some of us, caffeine aggravates teeth grinding. But add sugar and the tendency to sip beverages throughout the day, and you've created an environment perfect for tooth and root decay—to say nothing of diabetes and other obesity-related illness.

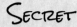

The good

So what's good about caffeine? Well, on its own it's low in calories—until you add sugar or cream. Then it's no longer a low-cal beverage.

Coffee is also the primary source of antioxidants for Americans, according to researchers at the University of Scranton. That's true whether the coffee is caffeinated or not—and the benefits extend only to a couple of cups a day.

Coffee has been associated with other benefits, including a lowered risk of type 2 diabetes. A recent study by the Harvard School of Public Health showed that increasing daily consumption by more than one cup a day over a four-year period lowered risk of developing type 2 diabetes by 11 percent. Decreasing consumption by the same amount increased risk by 17 percent. Oddly the results were true for coffee but not for tea.

An earlier study at the Harvard School of Public Health focused on the relationship between drinking coffee and death in 130,000 study volunteers. After 18 to 24 years, the researchers did not find an increased risk of death from any cause, including cancer or cardiovascular disease. That was true for people drinking up to six cups of coffee per day. But note that a cup of coffee was defined as 8 ounces with 100 mg of caffeine—not a Starbucks 16 ounce Grande or Pike's Place Roast with 330 mg of caffeine.

Caffeine has also been shown to improve athletic performance in sprints and endurance activities lasting up to two hours, according to Alex Hutchison, Ph.D., writing in *Which Comes First, Cardio or Weights?* In fact, caffeine was listed by the World Anti-Doping Association as a controlled or restricted substance until 2004 and the National Collegiate Athletic Association still lists it.

And that underscores a point that coffee drinkers often miss: Caffeine is a stimulant and a stimulant is a drug. And like most drugs, the effects are both good and bad.

The bad

Face it: If you drink coffee, one of the main reasons is probably its ability to wake you from the stupor of sleep and let you go about your day.

How does coffee get its ability to keep us awake? Caffeine blocks the hypnotic effect of adenosine, our bodies' natural sleeping pill, to keep us from falling asleep. In doing so, it helps us override our natural circadian rhythm, the wake-sleep cycle that is hardwired into each of us.

But this wakefulness comes at a price. When we don't get our required sleep, on average about eight hours, our bodies malfunction, physically, mentally and emotionally. Scientists already tell us that the United States is a sleep-deprived nation. But the answer to a chaotic lifestyle and busy schedule should not be an alarm clock and a caffeinated beverage—it should be more sleep.

Besides temporarily waking us, what else does caffeine do? It increases blood pressure, irritates the stomach lining, speeds digestion and causes heart palpitations.

And if you're drinking coffee every day, you're most likely addicted to caffeine. No, you're probably not going to go on a crime spree or engage in aberrant behavior, but you're still addicted.

Research from the Departments of Psychiatry and Neuroscience at Johns Hopkins Medical School reveals that people who take in only 100 mg of caffeine a day—that's one to two cups of coffee—can develop a physical dependence that results in withdrawal symptoms.

What are these symptoms? Headaches, muscle pain, stiffness, lethargy, nausea, vomiting, depression and irritability—although maybe not all at once. Withdrawal occurs from 12 to 24 hours after your last sip and can last as long as nine days. Chronic use of caffeine increases your tolerance and your withdrawal symptoms. If you are addicted, you already know this.

The ugly

And now the worst news: Even more serious than caffeine addiction and withdrawal is caffeine intoxication. The threat now comes not from your daily latte, but from the consumption of energy shots and drinks. Between 2007 and 2011, the number of U.S. emergency department visits due to energy drink overdose doubled from 10,068 to 20,783. That's according to the U.S. Substance Abuse and Mental Health Services Administration.

The young adults, age 18 to 25, who are the targets of energy-drink marketing campaigns, don't realize how much more potent these drinks are than a standard cup of joe. For example, one 2-ounce bottle of 5-Hour Energy® shot contains a whopping 200 mg of caffeine. That's half the recommended maximum intake of 400 mg per day for the average person—in just two ounces. Down a few bottles and you won't have any trouble staying awake.

The super-packed energy-drink industry grew to the $12.5 billion dollar mark in 2012. Expanding at a fervent pace, sales are expected to almost double to $21.5 billion by 2017. The major players are Red Bull, Monster®, 5-Hour Energy and Rockstar.

Not only are energy drinks and shots accessible at nearly every convenience store and major retailer, they're marketed like sodas for flavor, color and fun. They are even pumped into smoothies and alcoholic beverages, a shot or two at a time. Dr. Susan practices near a major university and hears from her college party-er patients that the late-night cocktail of choice is Jagermeister®, Red Bull and Viagra®.

Like soda, there's no nutritional value in energy drinks. And the calories displace nutrient-rich ones you might consume in a healthier diet. If you're a parent, you should know that research continues into the adverse effects of caffeine on children under 18. Again, 73 percent of youngsters are currently downing caffeinated drinks every day.

Keep your kids healthy by monitoring their caffeine consumption and ensuring it stays at or near zero. Remember to walk the talk. Youngsters have all eyes on your behaviors and habits, so limit the amount of caffeine you drink to well below the recommended limit of 400 mg per day. You'll regain some sleep, cut your grocery bill and keep your oral and overall health on the right track.

Quickstart to health

1. Drink caffeine in moderation.

Your maximum recommended caffeine consumption is 400 mg per day—the amount in four 8-ounce cups of coffee.

2. Keep your kids' caffeine consumption at or near zero.

Research continues into the adverse effects of caffeine on children under 18. Coffee shops and energy drink manufacturers target young people as a way to increase sales. But the ill effects of caffeine may be particularly potent in children.

3. Don't substitute coffee for a healthy lifestyle.

If you're tired because you don't eat a nutritious diet or you don't get enough sleep, all the caffeine in a Starbucks quad venti won't help. Your body needs good fuel and adequate rest.

4. If you suffer from migraines, quit coffee.

If you are a regular migraine headache sufferer, it's probably best to avoid caffeine as a regular drink. If you self-prescribe a daily drug that influences the contraction and expansion of the brain blood vessels, it might just be triggering your headaches.

Chapter 46

PROCESSED FOOD: KEEPING YOU ALIVE BUT NOT WELL

From the chair

SINCE SHE WAS 3 YEARS OLD, KALEE HAS BEEN PART *of my dental practice, first as a patient and now, at 27, as a colleague—a dental hygienist with a budding teaching career in total health. As a kid she was a tall, willowy, smart tooth geek with meticulous oral hygiene. But her excellent brushing and flossing skills and lack of visible plaque didn't spare her from red, puffy, bleeding gums—the signs of chronic gingivitis. The inflammation worsened as KaLee reached late adolescence.*

By the time KaLee went to college, she'd developed some other ugly symptoms: bloating, diarrhea, significant weight gain, severe gut pain and depression. She could not lose the extra pounds—a sign of chronic system inflammation—and that frustrated her.

Stabbing gut pain eventually sent her to a hospital emergency room one day. A bright young doc suggested she might be suffering from gluten sensitivity. She encouraged a six-month gluten vacation to see how KaLee would respond. After only one week, KaLee had lost her gut pain and five pounds along with it. After two more weeks, no one in her dental hygiene class, including the instructors, could believe that her gingivitis was 90 percent healed. And the best part for KaLee was the return of her positive attitude. As her depression lifted and she lost another 65 pounds, her entire outlook changed.

All due to food.

For years, dentists and physicians looked at the problems you presented—whether you had gingivitis in your mouth or a stabbing pain in your gut—and treated you with the best tools and medications they had at the time. But they rarely looked at your total health or helped you examine the root cause of problems or the possible connections to your lifestyle.

This fix-it model works fine if you have a broken leg from an accident. But it fails when your health is declining or you're aging—if you have gum disease, inflamed arteries, brain degeneration or a soft penis. Then you need a whole-

245

person approach to healthcare. A major part of that is examining what you're eating—and also what you're *not* eating.

In a healthy state, every part of our bodies, from our individual cells to our psychological state, has an intrinsic ability to heal—until it doesn't. By the time we feel sick, sluggish, fuzzy or sad, we have already suffered significant cell damage. And like KaLee, we may simply forget what healthy feels like. But what does it take to put all our cells in a position to heal and fend off other threats?

One critical ingredient is nutrient-dense whole foods.

Too many Americans eat much too much of another food group: junk. Instead of whole food, millions turn to flour-sugar-salt-chemical-laden foods. In fact, the Center for Nutrition Policy and Promotion, part of the U.S. Department of Agriculture, reports that only 10 percent of Americans have a "good" diet.

Many health professionals, including Mary Beth Palmer-Gierlinger, the nutrition coach for Dr. Susan's dental practice, believe that the risks of junk food consumption go beyond the rise in the classic "big three" diseases: heart disease, cancer and diabetes. These foods may also be responsible, in large part, for the drastic increase in allergies and autoimmune conditions. At this point, three or four generations have relied on junk and processed food, making our typical American diet virtually unrecognizable to our great-grandparents.

Nutrient-dense whole foods require neither processing nor the addition of nutrients to boost their health value. You can choose from a range of lean proteins, accompanied by vegetables, beans, fruits, nuts and whole grains packed with fiber and micronutrients—the very ones we are lacking today. In processed foods the nutrient level has bottomed out, and the deficiency gets worse if junk becomes a habitual replacement for whole foods.

And that's exactly what's happened to the American diet as a whole. Research reported in March 2015 shows that highly processed foods make up more than 60 percent of the calories in foods Americans buy. These foods include soda, cookies, chips, white bread, candy and prepared meals. Food manufacturers may ultimately need incentives to improve the nutrient value of their products.

" SECRET

Highly processed foods contain more fat, sugar and salt than less-processed foods. To curb overeating and obesity, avoid any food in a bag or a box as well as ready-to-eat, ready-to-heat meals. "

Below you'll find nutrition recommendations from Dr. Susan and her certified health coach, Mary Beth Palmer-Gierlinger. Mary Beth was trained at the Institute for Integrative Nutrition and has studied more than 100 dietary theories with some of the world's top health and wellness experts. Here are recommendations they believe will make the greatest difference in your oral and whole-body health.

Quickstart to health

The big takeaways

1. Limit sugar consumption.

The World Health Organization recommends everyone limit total sugar intake to 5 percent or less of daily calories. An adult of average build consumes around 2,000 calories a day, so 5 percent represents 100 calories—about two-thirds of a can of soda—for the entire day. Learn more in Chapter 43, Sugar.

2. Cut flour consumption.

In a recent interview, Dr. Steven Masley, former director of the Pritikin Longevity Center and author of the book *10 Years Younger*, explained that flour provokes the same chemical response in your bloodstream as sugar does—which could increase your risk of developing metabolic syndrome. What's metabolic syndrome? It's a group of risk factors for heart disease and type 2 diabetes, including high blood pressure, blood sugar and cholesterol, plus excess abdominal fat.

3. Cut hydrogenated fat consumption.

These solid fats extend a food's shelf life, but they will shorten your own life by increasing your risk of heart attack, stroke and cancer. Although most of us know we should avoid hydrogenated fats, we may not realize we're eating them in processed, packaged or restaurant foods. And we may not recognize the names for these dangerous fats in ingredient lists. Substitute with the healthy fats we list in "The Big Add-ons."

4. Consider cutting gluten.

Gluten is a protein locked into wheat, barley and rye. Even if you don't have the rare gluten-intolerant condition of celiac disease, you may be among the 6 to 20 percent of U.S. adults who are sensitive to these grains and their byproducts. Try a 21-day gluten vacation. Or if you want a sensitivity test without changing your diet, get one through Cyrex™ lab for about $350.

5. Consider cutting dairy.

About 10 percent of us are sensitive to dairy lactose, which can cause inflammatory gut symptoms similar to those for gluten sensitivity. If you suspect you're sensitive, try the same 21-day "cleanse" as above and see how your body responds.

6. Consider cutting other common pro-inflammatory foods.

If you still suffer from inflammation, consider taking a vacation from animal flesh, nuts (especially peanuts), soy products, corn and nightshade vegetables, including peppers, tomatoes, eggplant and potatoes.

7. Limit your exposure to toxins.

Nix all artificial sweeteners, preservatives, food additives and flavor enhancers. Read labels: If it doesn't sound like food, it's not. You may also want to choose organic foods, because pesticides, herbicides and antibiotics in the conventional food system get deposited in our body fat and have a strong correlation to cancer and other inflammatory disease. And, if you eat animal proteins, make sure the animals and their dairy-giving sisters have been eating organic too.

The big add-ons

Taking away foods that limit your health is only half the equation. You may also be suffering from nutritional deficiencies. Filling these can be a tall order, but you can start by increasing fruits and vegetables or by adding high-quality plant-derived supplements.

1. Add fiber—especially soluble fiber.

Most of us are deficient in fiber—the essence of fruits, veggies, nuts and beans. Fiber can tame the insulin spike that results from excessive sugar consumption and lower your risk of developing type 2 diabetes, as discussed in Chapter 14. According to the Institute of Medicine, adult women need 25 grams of fiber a day and men need 38 grams. Dr. Masley recommends that adults aim for 50 grams. In addition, he suggests that two-thirds of that be from soluble fiber from vegetables, fruits, beans and nuts.

2. Get adequate Vitamin D.

Most of us are deficient in Vitamin D, which can be serious because it compromises our immunity. Vitamin D comes in two forms, D2 and D3. D2 comes from plant foods; D3 comes from animal foods, such as fish, eggs and liver, *and* your body also produces it when your skin is exposed to a big dose of sunshine. How well we absorb it from food varies a lot depending on our age, lifestyle and health, so there is no one-size-fits-all prescription for getting up to healthy levels. The Vitamin D Council recommends we take 2,000 IU daily if we get little sun, although for deficiency your wellness doctor may recommend 5,000 to 10,000 IU of D3 for a month or so until you get up to par.

3. Eat healthy fats and omega 3 fats.

Many of us are deceived into thinking that refined junk oils from genetically modified plants like corn and canola qualify as "healthy." Nope. Get healthy omega 3 fats from fish, flax seed or flax oil, olive oil, coconut oil, avocado, nuts and seeds. Eating them daily lowers inflammation, depression and heart-threatening triglycerides, and supports brain health.

4. Boost antioxidants.

These healthy cell protectors and cancer-cell blockers come mostly from plants like brightly colored berries, legumes, dark greens like kale, sweet potatoes, dark grapes like the ones in wine, plus a variety of other fruits and vegetables with deep color. Bonus: All of these are also packed with fiber.

5. Eat lean and plant-based protein.

Most wellness docs and nutritionists say Americans consume too much protein. Remember that extra protein will *not* help you build more muscle or gain strength—what cannot be used for energy right away is stored as fat. Check the USDA guidelines to see how much protein you need every day. And protein doesn't need to be meat. Some of the best protein sources come from plants, such as legumes of all kinds, seeds, nuts and whole grains. Also consider seafood like small-mouth, wild-caught fish and lean, protein-rich, animal-based proteins, such as eggs and Greek yogurt.

6. Choose whole grains.

Whole grains have not been polished, stripped or ground, so 100 percent of the original kernel (the bran, germ and endosperm) is present. These are high in fiber and protein but are also nutrient-rich. Whole grains come in a variety of tastes and textures, including quinoa, wild rice, brown rice, oats, barley, cracked wheat, bulgur and wheatberries.

7. Consume magnesium-rich foods.

Magnesium is a chemical element found in more than 300 different enzymes in your body. Turns out it's a key player in removing toxins from your body—and thereby helping you to prevent cell damage from dangerous environmental chemicals and heavy metals. Magnesium also plays a major role in reducing stress and managing weight. You'll find it in dark leafy greens, nuts, seeds, fish, beans, avocados and whole grains—and dark chocolate.

8. Eat calcium-rich foods.

We always associate calcium with strong bones and teeth, and it does help prevent osteoporosis. Calcium also helps regulate muscle contractions and prevent heart disease and certain types of cancer. In addition to milk and yogurt, other foods rich in calcium include leafy greens like kale and spinach, legumes, some fruits, and seafood like sardines.

9. Consume cruciferous vegetables.

Cruciferous vegetables have it all: fiber, phytochemicals, vitamins, minerals and antioxidants. Eat at least a cup a day of broccoli, cauliflower, Brussels sprouts, kale, cabbage or bok choy. They will enhance your liver's ability to detox your body and help lower your risk of cancer, heart disease and stroke.

10. Drink healthy beverages.

Start with water, water and more water. The Institute of Medicine's general guidelines suggest 125 ounces (about 15 cups) for men and 91 ounces (about 11 cups) for women every day. If you like lemon water, limit it to mealtimes, because it can cause acid erosion of the enamel on your teeth. Drink tea and coffee in moderation, but cut back on fruit juices and milk—and totally cut out real or artificially sweetened beverages. Limit alcohol to one serving per day if you're a woman, two if you're a man.

SECTION 12

THE HEALTHY PRACTICE

The significant mouth-body connections we've highlighted throughout **BlabberMouth!** make it clear that oral health has a deep impact on total health. That means your dentist plays an ever-more critical role in ensuring you live a healthy, happy, sexy—and long—life. But that requires a new model for dental care, one that focuses on far more than your teeth and gums. So what should you look for in the healthy dental practice?

Start by choosing a healthcare team that will work *with* you, not just *on* you. This approach goes far beyond sick care at your physician or a quick pop-in by your dentist after your regular exam. In Chapter 47, The High-Touch Practice, we'll talk about putting together a team you can partner with to achieve an optimal state of health and wellness.

To be most effective, the new model of dental care requires advanced technology—from electronic health records that can be easily shared to screening tools that can quickly identify disease. We'll tell you about new tools that give your team more time to establish a meaningful relationship with you in Chapter 48, The High-Tech Practice.

Of course, you'll always get your teeth cleaned prior to a dental exam. But Chapter 49, Clean Thoroughly, Polish Selectively, explains that even some procedures you take for granted have changed. The reason: As research brings to light new information on the best treatments for your mouth, your dentist should change how she practices to incorporate that knowledge.

We'll discuss one innovation that may be coming to your dental practice—if it hasn't already arrived—in Chapter 50, Salivary Diagnostics. Throughout **BlabberMouth!**, we've talked about the mouth as a window to the body—and that makes the dental office the ideal setting to perform initial screenings for systemic diseases, such as diabetes and human papillomavirus, and further diagnostics that cover every aspect of oral and systemic health.

In Chapter 51, Exam Time, you'll discover how the twice-a-year dental exam differs in a progressive dental practice that understands oral-systemic health.

251

Your dentist and hygienist look at your teeth and gums, sure, but they also evaluate how your oral health could impact your risk of diseases from heart disease, diabetes and pregnancy complications to depression and sexual issues.

Chapter 47

THE HIGH-TOUCH PRACTICE: BUILDING YOUR TEAM

AS OF 2012, about half of all adults in the United States—some 117 million people—suffer from one or more chronic health conditions, according to the Centers for Disease Control. One-quarter of those individuals have two or more chronic health conditions.

And yet, according to a 2013 survey by the American Academy of Family Physicians, the average primary-care doc is responsible for a whopping 2,367 patients—and sees just around 100 of them every week.

It's not unusual for visits to a physician to be scheduled in 15-minute intervals, which leaves even less time for a face-to-face consultation with you. Your physician may have only enough time to address your chief concern—heartburn, trouble sleeping, a sore throat—and to write a prescription for your symptoms. The rapid turnaround simply won't allow a discussion of lifestyle changes that might resolve the underlying issues. The result? Your physician feels like a hamster on a wheel and you feel rushed and unheard.

The same scenario may play out with your dentist, as he moves from one treatment room to the next, filling a cavity in one, consulting on tooth lightening in another and dropping in at the end of a cleaning to do a quick exam in a third.

And yet being heard and feeling cared for is critical to your well-being. Studies reported during the past 30 years show that a physician's ability to explain, listen and empathize can have a profound impact on both biological and functional health outcomes—and on your satisfaction and experience of the care provided.

As you become more educated on health and more aware of your own needs, you may realize you want a physician or dentist who doesn't run an assembly line or follow a cookie-cutter philosophy when it comes to treatment. But that will require you to establish specific criteria for what you want—and to conduct a search to find the right players for your healthcare team.

The must-have criteria

So how should you put together a dream healthcare team, whether you're looking for a dentist, physician or specialist?

1. Get recommendations. Start by asking your family or friends, but be certain you know why a provider prompts enthusiasm. A warm personality is definitely a plus, but it must be matched by clinical expertise. You may also want to check the web to identify prospects. You can get a feel for the physician's or dentist's office, values, practice philosophies and expertise or emphasis. You'll also find out if the provider is available by email or phone or takes calls from established patients on weekends.

2. Don't feel trapped by your insurance plan. Yes, you'll want to find out if a practice honors your current insurance plan—and what the payment options and financial obligations might be. But also expand your search to include practices that may be out of your network. You might be pleasantly surprised that the added value is far greater than your added cost.

3. Interview candidates. Once you've identified a few candidates, set up a call or visit to get to know the physician or dentist. Most will be happy to talk with you for a few moments. Learn about the office culture, the pace of visits and the physician's patience with people who want a shared discussion. Ask as many questions as you need to determine if you are a fit for each other. If you don't feel comfortable with the initial interview or if the office doesn't have the time, knowledge or interest to answer your questions, move on.

4. Make sure your approaches and goals align. Healthcare providers and their teams vary a great deal in their philosophical approach to patients. The relationships you choose should be collaborative, meaning your opinions matter. The days of the patriarchal medical model, where the father-like physician determines the diagnosis and tells the patient exactly what to do, are gone—or they should be. You want a dentist or physician who is curious about where you've been, where you are and what health goals you are striving for. You want your story and ideas to influence the physician's treatment recommendations.

5. Expect generosity of time. Two-way dialogue generally takes more than a brief visit with your physician or a pop-in by your dentist. That doesn't build a solid doctor-patient relationship. You don't want to leave with a prescription when what you really need is help to identify the root cause and change your health habits. Your own curiosity should be respected too—you don't want to feel stupid or rushed because you ask questions that require in-depth answers.

6. Check for clinical expertise. Yes, you definitely want a physician or dentist who attended a solid medical or dental school. But "board certification" in a specialty requires higher training and extra exams with continued renewal, which all tell you your doctor is serious about giving patients the benefit of advanced knowledge.

7. Look for perpetual learners. New understandings in dentistry and medicine are continually unfolding, so the most responsible docs never stop learning. To practice based on the most recent and applicable research findings—known as evidence-based practice—requires dedication to high-level learning, a constant eye on newly published studies, flexibility to change current practices and humility to explain to patients why the new approach beats the old one. Don't be afraid to ask your docs what they do to keep up with the rapidly growing body of medical and dental knowledge.

8. Treat your body as a whole. Look for physicians and dentists who favor a thorough and comprehensive approach rather than focusing on one ailment at a time. There is a growing demand for care teams who look at you as a whole, including your lifestyle, and help you develop optimal function of all your organs. Many patients are also considering programs that offer comprehensive preventive and diagnostic exams all in one place.

9. Be patient. Be aware that if you do find a physician or dentist who encourages dialogue with patients, he may struggle to stay on schedule. Make sure you're willing to wait a few minutes to accommodate his need to make time to talk to all his patients about their concerns.

10. Balance high-tech and high-touch. You will reap many benefits if your healthcare team is incorporating the latest high-tech equipment and services in their practices. But the technology should be matched by an equal share of wholehearted human connection.

> ## Secret
>
> When you are choosing a healthcare provider of any kind, remember that it's your body, your time and your money. But also know that if you're health-aware, you always have your own personal physician at hand—you.

Preparing for a visit

Once you find a physician or dentist or other provider for your healthcare team, remember that you're part of the team too. To make the most of every appointment, prepare in advance.

1. Do some research. Run an online search of your symptoms, making sure you choose legitimate health sources like WebMD or Mayo Clinic. Showing up to your doctor's visit with some common language and hunches about what's going on is helpful—and it shows your level of concern and commitment to a good outcome. But don't be a know-it-all. Let your docs follow their educated, experienced suspicions and order appropriate diagnostic tests.

2. Know your history. Keep a written log of your symptoms, incidents, diagnoses, treatment recommendations and medications. This helps make your visit more effective, because you won't waste time recalling specifics, while potentially sacrificing accuracy.

3. Follow up as directed. When your doctor recommends tests or specialists, ask what you can expect. To increase your understanding, schedule a follow-up appointment to discuss test results rather than waiting for an office administrator to write or call back with results.

4. Ask your dentist and physicians to bridge the gaps. Many times we have multiple providers addressing different problems, each prescribing different medications that may have unhealthy interactions when taken together. No body system is isolated from the others. So it's safe to assume that all your oral and systemic issues are related in some way, and that all your dental and medical providers will benefit from a look at the overall picture. Systemic health concerns associated with poor oral health, including diabetes, high blood pressure, cancer and multiple prescription medications, make a collaborative approach even more critical.

5. Provide feedback to improve care. Most of us like to be recognized when we walk into our doctors' offices, especially if we are seeking a little extra

TLC for an urgent situation. That special attention is why many patients enjoy the friendly, personal feel of the smaller dental office. But even a practice that strives to be high-touch can fall short of the mark. When Dr. Susan's dental team was switching from paper to electronic health records, the frustrating process sometimes distracted her staff from warm, present, personal communications. That brings up a key point: If you're ever feeling slighted or disappointed by your treatment, don't be afraid to provide some gentle feedback to your physician or dentist. Your words could serve as a helpful wake-up call.

Remember: There's little more important to the quality and even the quantity of your life than your health. It's worthwhile to be truly discerning in finding partners you trust to collaborate on your health goals. Be patient and persistent— you deserve the best.

Quickstart to health

1. Consider carefully the key characteristics for your healthcare team.

Make a list of all the must-haves and good-to-haves important to you in your physician or dentist, from clinical expertise, board certifications and continuing education to personality, payment options, insurance accepted and languages spoken.

2. Get recommendations from referring doctors, friends and family.

Don't just take names and numbers; also dig deeper to find out *why* an individual recommends a particular healthcare provider for you in particular.

3. Check out websites to learn about candidates.

The physician's or dentist's website will give you information about their expertise, advanced training, communication style, values and practice.

4. Interview candidates by phone or in person.

If you want a collaborator, make sure the physician or dentist honors your role and works *with* you to ensure optimal oral and overall health for yourself.

5. Use appointment time efficiently.

Do some research on your symptoms online and make sure you keep a detailed health history. Then follow up if your dentist or physician recommends tests or consultations with specialists.

Chapter 48

The High-Tech Practice: For the Patients' Benefit

Diana

"She's doing great, isn't she?" *My hygienist, Cezanne, was wrapping up her exam with a verbal hand-off to my dentist, Dr. Duke.*

He'd followed up her exam with one of his own. Now we were reviewing my digital x-rays on the exam room's screen while Cezanne took notes on a chairside computer. Just a few years before, when Dr. Duke started his practice, he still used the old film-and-lightbox x-ray technology. But I recall his excitement two years ago, when he told me his plans for remodeling the building and, more importantly, for updating the practice's technology.

Now he pondered a lower right molar on the screen. "This tooth worries me. It looks like a compass, with fractures heading off in all four directions. If it breaks, you could need a root canal or even an implant. I'd like to replace that filling with a crown."

*We'd had this discussion several years prior. At the time, I wasn't particularly worried about fractures in my teeth—but that was in my pre-***BlabberMouth!*** days.*

"Four factures in one tooth? What does it look like?" *I asked.*

Dr. Duke whipped out a pen that turned out to be a camera. Just 30 seconds later, my cracked-up molar appeared in high definition, much larger than life.

"You've made your point," *I said.* "I'll schedule an appointment."

> **" Secret**
>
> High-tech diagnostic equipment exists to serve you, the patient, with a more precise diagnosis and better understanding of your condition. Use it as a springboard for discussions that will help you make more informed treatment decisions. **"**

Like Dr. Susan's and Dr. Duke's practice, 59 percent of U.S. dental offices are solo or small group practices. And many offer new technology that supports advanced dental treatment and cosmetic enhancement.

But the expense of high-tech equipment also means that dentists are banding together to share facilities, equipment—and costs. From the patient standpoint, the greater convenience could be good. For instance, if your dentist refers you to a "blank-o-dontist"—and by that we mean an orthodontist, periodontist, endodontist, prosthodontist, pediatric dentist or oral surgeon—it's easier if they're in-house or next door. If you survey patients, many say they would rather be treated under the same roof than referred across town.

The key? High-tech advances should benefit you, not just the practice, by improving patient-dentist communication, broadening treatment options and decreasing exposure to harmful substances.

Let's take a look at just some of the types of specialty equipment your dentist may be using to enhance your treatment.

Digital photography: To capture images of your face or the inside of your mouth and show them to you on a monitor, most dentists use a camera. The *intra-oral* camera, which Dr. Duke used to capture an image of Diana's molar, is a small, pen-sized wand with a flexible range of focus. Your dentist can maneuver it to capture images inside your mouth and show large-size versions on-screen.

Extra-oral photographs are taken from outside your mouth with special lenses that capture detail on a larger scale. These pics generally require the use of retractors. Retractors move your cheeks out of the way; along with mirrors, they can reflect an entire arch in one photo.

All these images provide excellent communication tools, allowing better understanding of what's going on inside and outside your mouth. They also improve collaboration when you discuss treatment options with your dentist.

Digital x-rays: If you're worried about cumulative radiation or are done with holding strange configurations of cardboard in your mouth, then you'll be delighted with digital x-rays. In just a few seconds, an intra-oral sensor captures ultra-detailed images, with about 90 percent less radiation than the traditional approach. Extra-oral sensors produce the Panorex x-ray, which zooms around your head, and also provides more thorough images with less radiation than ever before.

Computed tomography (CT) scans: A growing trend among dentists is a high-tech imaging system called CBCT (cone beam computed tomography) that captures a three-dimensional image of an area of the mouth. These are especially helpful in planning dental implant placement—the surgeon can see the configuration of bone and choose the exact size and angle of the implant placement. CT is also used to plan precision orthodontic outcomes and scan for lesions, such as cysts, abscesses or cancers.

Chairside computers: Many dentists have installed computing equipment in treatment rooms to help with data collection, record keeping and patient communication. A large portion of dentists will soon run "paperless" offices to comply with the demand for electronic health record sharing.

Computer-aided design (CAD)/computer-aided machining (CAM) restorative solutions: A growing trend in the high-tech dental office is to do away with goopy impressions and temporary crowns. Now it's possible to use a scanning device to take a specialized picture of a prepared tooth—one that has been shaped for a large filling, crown or veneer. Then the data are used to create a virtual 3-D model instead of a plaster model. The dentist can send the virtual model electronically to a dental laboratory to produce a tooth-colored restoration. Or the restoration can be milled right in the office. These expensive and tech-sexy milling machines have become more and more common in mainstream dentistry.

Laser dentistry: Diagnostic lasers let dentists detect cavities much sooner than with x-rays and exams. That's a great plus for preventive dentistry. Dentists can also use surgical lasers for many soft-tissue surgeries, including reshaping gums or relieving babies of a "tongue-tied" condition, so infants can latch on for breast feeding. These surgeries can even be done without numbing—and with little bleeding or discomfort. Some lasers are also used to cut hard tissue for applications such as preparing teeth for restorations.

Quickstart to health

1. Recognize the value of high-tech equipment or an expanded practice.

Most dental teams are excited about offering technology they believe can improve your care. Ask about your dentist's latest investments in technology to keep yourself up-to-date on what's available to you and why.

2. Understand that some dentists may join a group to share the cost of new equipment and facilities.

Some patients prefer a smaller, more intimate office; others appreciate the convenience of a one-stop shop that includes multiple dental practitioners with varied expertise. Be flexible about the one best for you—if your long-time dentist joins a partnership or group, the practice may still provide the friendly, personal treatment you prefer.

Chapter 49

CLEAN THOROUGHLY, POLISH SELECTIVELY: THE NEW HEALTHY

YOU CALL IT A CLEANING; your dentist and hygienist call it *prophylaxis*. That sounds daunting, until you remember that another name for condom is *prophylactic*—a different kind of prevention, but prevention nonetheless. Dental prophylaxis, or "prophy" for short, is a preventive cleaning to fend off dental diseases—including tooth decay and gum disease—and associated systemic diseases as well.

Until recently, cleaning was always followed up with polishing. But in evidence-based dental practices, that may no longer be the case. Why not? Stay with us and we'll tell you why research says you should be selective about treatments that abrade your teeth.

The cleaning

Preventing gum disease takes a multifaceted approach, but certainly one key element is getting the *gak* off your teeth. "Gak" is a facetious term coined by Dr. Susan's team to describe the whole plaque-tartar combo. "De-gak-ing" refers to scraping and flushing the big stuff.

Keep in mind that preventing disease is not the same thing as treating disease. In fact the prophy is defined as *an above-the gumline cleaning in the absence of inflammation.* That means your hygienist cleans your teeth from your biting surfaces down to your gum border—and not below. So before your prophy, she should measure your pocket depths and look for bone loss and especially bleeding, the #1 sign of active inflammation.

Dental hygienists are notoriously driven to scrape off all the calcified plaque—called calculus or tartar—both above *and* below the gumline, often treating active gum disease under the guise of a regular prophy.

261

If your hygienist or dentist probes deeper pockets in your gums and finds active inflammation, you will need a more targeted kind of cleaning—one that extends to *subgingival*, which are sites below the gumline. Both periodontal treatment and periodontal maintenance cleanings require more advanced skills and time. That's because the hygienist is now working on areas not visible to her, using site-specific instruments and often local anesthesia to ease gum and root-surface sensitivity.

If you previously have had gum disease and are left with residual pockets, you need a *periodontal maintenance prophy*. Bone lost around your teeth doesn't grow back—so even if deeper pockets don't bleed when cleaning them, they require more care and attention from your hygienist. Accessing the deepest part of these residual pockets is difficult—or even impossible—for you to do at home. Research suggests that for maintenance, three-month professional cleanings are optimal.

The not-so-shiny truth about polishing

If you're old enough to be reading this, then you're probably old enough to recall having all of your teeth polished after the scraping was done. That may have happened even at your last appointment.

Mmmmm, said your tongue, after the hygienist finished. *So slick, so slippery, so smo-o-o-o-th.*

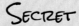

And for about an hour, your mouth felt cleaner than ever. But sooner than you can say "biofilm," the layer called that (or sometimes *pellicle*) re-grew on your teeth. And that's a good thing, because ultimately it provides your teeth with a thin cloak of protection.

Turns out that polishing is not so good for your teeth—and that's been known for years. *Selective polishing for stain*—and stain alone—is preached in dental schools and dental hygiene schools around the country.

" SECRET

Multiple studies show that polishing teeth with a rubber cup and gritty paste can cause abrasion and should be performed selectively, for unsightly stain only. It's not effective for preventing cavities or gingivitis. **"**

That's even a secret for many dental teams, who cling to the status quo. Dr. Susan realizes that the dentists and hygienists who do know this and polish anyway, do it because they don't want to disappoint you. You need to trust the research and be satisfied with a professional cleaning that does not include abrasive polishing.

Why? Picture your teeth under a microscope. Enamel is like a massive stack of glass tubules—tiny straws arranged perpendicular to the surface. They suck up whatever moisture they touch. Maybe it's saliva, which is perfect, or maybe it's juice-soda-sports drinks-energy drinks, which are not so perfect because they're all highly acidic. In fact, if you add that acid to the acid produced by sugar-eating bacteria in your plaque, the glassy enamel tubules start to dissolve.

The solution? Topical fluoride from toothpaste, rinses, professionally applied gels or, best of all, professionally applied fluoride varnishes. The fluoride molecule acts like Elmer's® glue, clogging the glass-like tubules. Clogging sounds bad, but in this case clogging protects the tooth from absorbing these harmful acids. Of course, fluoride must be continually reapplied to reinforce its protective power.

Here's the rub about polishing teeth: Polishing with professional abrasive paste removes the biofilm *and* the fluoride-protected layer of enamel. Abrasion is even more harmful for kids, because the enamel on baby teeth is far thinner.

And that fluoride-rich layer won't come back right away. In fact, it can take up to three months to rebuild the cavity protection and erase the sensitivity to cold, heat and touch. Polishing actually harms the tooth.

Could it get any worse? Why yes, it could. If you choose to have a fluoride varnish applied to your teeth, polishing off the biofilm beforehand makes that varnish a little less effective. The data say the intact biofilm acts as a scaffold to hold the fluoride on the enamel surface longer. The longer the fluoride stays there, the greater the penetration and the more effectively it prevents cavities.

A different option

You're probably familiar with this saying from a few centuries back: "Give a man a fish and you'll feed him for a day. Teach a man to fish and you'll feed him for a lifetime." Minus the fish, this principle can also apply to your dental cleaning appointment. Instead of polishing, Dr. Susan recommends that dental hygienists take the time they would spend on polishing to watch you brush and floss, and coach you toward a thorough plaque removal. Working on personal skill-building with each patient, especially children, is an investment in a lifetime of prevention and health.

If you're still getting a full polish, it's up to you to tell your dentist or hygienist that you'd prefer polish for visible stain only. And if you're even slightly cavity-prone, insist on leaving with fluoride varnish protection at each and every cleaning appointment.

Quickstart to health

1. Ask your hygienist and/or dentist to tell you about pockets and inflammation.

You want to be informed about gum disease and then work with your dentist and hygienist to address the causes and treatment.

2. If you have residual pockets, get a perio maintenance prophy.

A hygienist with advanced skills and special instruments needs to clean below the gumline in hard-to-reach areas to help prevent a resurgence of active gum disease.

3. Ask your hygienist to help you with personalized skill-building.

She can identify the areas you are missing with your toothbrush, floss or other cleaning widgets. Even better, she can teach you how to clean these tricky spots more effectively on your own.

4. Ask for polish only where stains are unsightly.

There's no point in removing the protein layer, called the biofilm, which helps fluoride protect your enamel longer. If you have surface stains, ask for just the ugly areas to be polished off with non-abrasive professional paste. Also consider more attention to your daily oral care.

5. Request a fluoride varnish if you're cavity-prone.

A fluoride varnish can give your teeth the added protection necessary to put a damper on decay.

Chapter 50

SALIVARY DIAGNOSTICS: THE SPITTING IMAGE OF YOUR HEALTH

FOR THE PAST SIX YEARS, the occurrence of oral cancer in the United States has continued to climb. But with an incidence rate that hovers around 3 percent, you probably wouldn't hear much about it, if it weren't for this: One in three Americans diagnosed with oral cancer dies within five years; many others are horribly disfigured. There's hope for changing these disheartening statistics, however—not just for oral cancer, but for many other diseases—and that hope depends on spit.

Let's look first at why an American dies of oral cancer about once an hour. Quite simply, it's just tough to diagnose the disease before it reaches an advanced stage. Most oral cancers are hidden in the tongue, floor of the mouth and throat, making them hard to detect even with oral cancer screenings. By the time the cancer is detected, it has often moved into the lymph nodes and metastasized. For a frightening example of how hard a tumor is to find even when the patient can tell you exactly where they're hurting, read actor Michael Douglas' story in Chapter 27, Oral Cancer.

Yes, illumination with fluorescent light and brush biopsies help. But the cancerous lesion must already be visible to diagnose it. That's often not the case in the early stages—and although that's an issue in the United States, it's absolutely critical in developing countries where the oral cancer incidence rates are much higher. In India, for example, oral cancer is the third most common, amounting to more than 30 percent of all malignancies in that country.

These challenges prompted researcher Dr. David Wong of the University of California Los Angeles and his colleagues to develop a saliva-based test to identify telltale signs of oral cancer. The telltale signs are biomarkers—RNA molecules, which make proteins that run our bodies, and the proteins themselves. These show consistently different levels in the saliva of individuals suffering from oral cancer.

Late in 2014, a small company called PeriRx announced a salivary diagnostic test for oral cancer based on Dr. Wong's work. The rinse-and-spit test is administered chairside, then sent to a lab for diagnosis. It's just one example from the exploding field of salivary diagnostics, a ray of hope for detecting and preventing disease and initiating treatment when it can do the most good.

SECRET

Early detection of disease drastically improves treatment outcomes. Saliva provides a rapid, noninvasive means to test for oral and systemic diseases. Soon your results will be analyzed and available right at the point of care.

Spit clues

Dozens of new saliva tests are quickly moving from laboratory technology to reality in clinical settings. High-tech instruments suck in saliva and spit out test results in a matter of minutes, right in the dental office or other nontraditional diagnostic setting.

Saliva offers unlimited potential as a diagnostic fluid, including advantages over blood, urine and other bodily fluids. Saliva collection is less expensive, less invasive, less cumbersome, painless and, yes, less embarrassing than other collection methods.

How does it work? Picture saliva as a gooey conglomeration of fluid, mixed with food, microorganisms and blood secretions. Want more detail? "Whole" saliva includes the fluid from the cuff of the gum tissue, blood serum, blood derivatives from mouth sores and inflamed gums, sloughed skin cells, bronchial and nasal secretions, bacteria and their byproducts, viruses, fungi and food debris. Sounds confusing and yucky, but from that scientists can unlock DNA/RNA, proteins, hormones, electrolytes, enzymes, antibodies and antimicrobial constituents specific to you. In fact, dentists refer to saliva as the "mirror of the body."

What disease markers can we now detect? Here's just a sampling—but remember, scientists are continually adding to the list:

• Bacteria, like the ones that cause cavities and periodontal disease;

• Viruses like HPV and human immunodeficiency virus (HIV);

• DNA/RNA biomarkers for many different early-stage organ and blood cancers;

• Inflammatory markers that predict heart disease or even indicate a recent heart attack;

- Autoimmune diseases, such as Sjögren's syndrome;

- Genetic disorders like cystic fibrosis and ectodermal dysplasia;

- A history of drug use.

In Dr. Susan's dental office today, you can not only be spit-tested for HPV infection, but you can also learn if you carry the gene that makes you prone to gum disease and heart disease—which will help you and your dentist and physicians make effective long-term treatment plans. Dr. Susan's practice offers another saliva test that identifies the DNA of the individual bacteria present in gum disease. By detecting the presence of the most dangerous bacteria, she can prescribe specific antibiotics in conjunction with conventional periodontal treatment and monitor post-treatment results with follow-up bacteria testing.

The future of spit testing

The National Institutes of Health (NIH) predict a future where salivary diagnostics will be used in everyday dental and medical situations. Imagine portable testing devices that are able to measure from one to possibly hundreds of compounds in saliva within minutes, all with an instrument about the size of a new iPhone®. Imagine the possibility of using just a single drop of saliva to provide early diagnosis for otherwise killer cancers—including pancreatic, liver, ovarian, lung, gastric, breast and oral cancer—and to design a targeted approach to treatment. These technologies lie within our grasp but will need to pass rigorous testing and approval for point-of-care use.

Spit can be used to provide information on your metabolic status too. If you need to call an ambulance for someone in your family, for instance, the emergency medical technician will soon be able to take a spit sample from the patient while under way and load it into a fully automated test cartridge. By the time the patient arrives at the hospital, extensive results based on the sample will already be available.

As scientists continue to miniaturize the technology, the NIH suggests it may someday be possible to attach a tiny device to your tooth and let you monitor medication levels and biomarkers for specific diseases.

Saliva tests may eventually prove to be inexpensive enough that they allow screening of a large population for both common and not-so-common diseases even before symptoms are seen. The tests support rapid communication and decision-making, faster start to effective treatment and monitoring for improvement—factors that may not lower the incidence of disease but should definitely impact the outcome.

Quickstart to health

1. Consider a saliva test for genetic predisposition to periodontal disease.

If positive, your dentist can use the results to customize your treatment plan and let your physician know you are also more prone to cardiovascular disease. Learn more about interleukin genetic testing in Chapter 11, Heart Disease, and Chapter 4, Periodontal Disease.

2. If you have periodontal disease, get a saliva test to identify the bacteria.

Your dentist will use the information to prescribe antibiotics specific to your infection and set you up for a post-treatment follow-up test.

3. If you have not been vaccinated for HPV, consider a saliva test for persistent infection.

Learn more about HPV infection and its associated oral cancer risk in Chapter 27, Oral Cancer.

4. Stay tuned.

Point-of-care salivary diagnostics will soon be available in your dental office, at your regular cleaning and exam appointment.

Chapter 51

Exam Time:
The Dental Visit Reimagined

DURING A DENTAL VISIT just 50 years ago, your hygienist cleaned your teeth, took cavity-detecting x-rays and then stepped aside as the dentist performed a simple dental exam—a look at your teeth.

Today we can all but guarantee that your visit will include a health history review, oral cancer screening and gum exam. But given that your oral health can be critical for your long-term overall health, your dental exam may soon be even more comprehensive. That starts with an expanded role for your dental hygienist.

> ## Secret
>
> Your hygienist is often the only healthcare provider you see for a regularly scheduled preventive visit. Your hygienist and dentist can serve as early detectors of systemic disease, as well as dedicated health advocates to manage communications and care with other health professionals.

If your hygienist and your dentist are progressive, they truly want to understand how your oral health fits into your overall well-being and what risk factors you have for systemic disease. The practice may already be using high-tech diagnostic equipment, saliva testing and a much more collaborative approach to treat you. Given these advances, how could your dental exam look in the not-distant-at-all future?

How the future looks

Allan arrives for his 6-month dental appointment. His hygienist, Georgette, greets him warmly. She hands Allan an electronic tablet containing his health history from six months prior and asks him for an update.

Allan reports that he has had a recent unexplainable weight loss and an increase in his blood pressure medicine. Looking at his dental history, he tells Georgette about a swollen lymph node that recently appeared at the corner of his lower jaw. He also reports that he may have more bleeding than normal when he brushes and flosses. Georgette immediately incorporates Allan's updates into his electronic medical record.

The dialogue continues as Georgette asks about other unusual signs and symptoms. Allan's unexplained weight loss and bleeding gums prompt Georgette to suggest he take the self-screen risk assessment for diabetes (presented in Chapter 14, Diabetes). Allan scores high enough that Georgette recommends an A1C fingerstick blood test. The test provides information about blood sugar levels over the past three months.

Six minutes later, Georgette has a verdict: Allan has an A1C of 7.2, which falls in the range for type 2 diabetes. For a few minutes, the two discuss Allan's drive-thru eating habits and lack of exercise as possible contributors. Allan is justifiably concerned and vows to quit power-drinking soda. He also decides to schedule an appointment with Jean, the practice's health relationship coordinator, to discuss nutrition coaching. At the end of the appointment, Georgette and Dr. Susan will refer Allan to his physician for help with blood sugar control, including possible medication.

Next Georgette takes Allan's blood pressure to see if his change in medication is working. At 130/90, Allan's blood pressure is still elevated. Georgette makes a note to include that information in the letter Dr. Susan will send to Allan's prescribing physician.

Georgette tips the chair back and begins the physical exam with an oral cancer screening. She feels the node that Allan mentioned. Georgette explores his mouth for diseased teeth that may be the cause. Finding nothing out of the ordinary, Georgette suggests using a specialized oral cancer screening light that illuminates suspect tissue with fluorescent light.

Georgette sees what appears to be a dark area near Allan's right tonsil. After consulting with Dr. Susan, Georgette administers a saliva test for human papillomavirus (HPV) to determine if Allan might have a persistent infection that could pose an oral cancer risk. Dr. Susan also performs a brush biopsy of the at-risk tissue to check it at a cellular level. The prospect of oral cancer scares Allan, so Georgette talks with him matter-of-factly about the disease and his risk. When Allan is ready, the exam proceeds.

Next Georgette completes a temporomandibular joint (TMJ) screening and gives Allan the good news that all is within normal limits. Then she performs a perio exam. Allan was correct: His bleeding on probing scores are much higher than at his last visit. Georgette suggests that this might improve when his blood sugar returns to normal. In the meantime, Georgette strongly recommends site-specific periodontal therapy for four back teeth, where Allan's bone loss has advanced. Georgette suggests that before that visit, they perform a different saliva test to determine which bacteria are present, so Dr. Susan can select targeted antibiotics.

By now, Allan's scheduled visit is almost up. Dr. Susan joins them and conducts a second exam of Allan's mouth, while Georgette brings her up-to-date on her findings and discussion with Allan. Dr. Susan confirms the findings and electronically dictates all the communication points she wants to note for Allan's primary physician. The dictation is sent to Jean, who will draft a letter for Dr. Susan's review and signature.

Allan then sets up his next appointment with Georgette and Dr. Susan. At that appointment, they will provide the results of his brush biopsy and HPV saliva test, re-check his lymph node and take his blood pressure again. Another saliva test will help identify bacteria, which could make Allan more at risk for gum disease, as well as heart attack and stroke. If Allan's mouth contains threatening bacteria, Dr. Susan will write a prescription for the specific antibiotics needed, in conjunction with his site-specific periodontal cleaning.

Georgette and Dr. Susan both know that the threat of a positive cancer biopsy will cause Allan a great deal of stress over the next week. They reassure him that if he does have abnormal cells, they will work with him for the best possible treatment outcome.

Later that day, Jean will study all the exam notes along with Dr. Susan's electronic dictation. She will draft a letter to Allan's physician discussing his oral cancer examination, HPV saliva testing, diabetes diagnosis, blood pressure reading, exercise and diet counseling, active gum disease and plans for further diagnostic testing and treatment. This letter is only the first in a line of communications between Allan's dental and medical teams, who will work together to help him achieve total wellness.

Allan leaves the office, nervous but reassured by the expertise and the advocacy role of his dental team. He also knows he will have compassionate and continuing care. That's essential for him. Although Allan did not get his teeth cleaned today, he actually got much more—a personalized approach to his total health.

Quickstart to health

1. See your dentist at least twice a year.

This should be a comprehensive examination. Think of your semi-annual appointment as an investment in your total health, not just as a "cleaning."

2. Be thorough about your medical and dental history.

Tell your dental team about your complete medical history. Don't skip or gloss over parts you think have nothing to do with dental health. Studies increasingly show links between oral health and every part of the body.

3. Ask all your questions about your oral and total health.

Try to keep a running list of your oral health issues on your cell phone's note app. That way you'll be ready for your next preventive appointment. Also ask questions about your overall health and risk factors created or made worse by your oral health.

4. Expect a thorough assessment of oral and overall health risk factors.

Don't be surprised if your dentist discusses topics that seem unrelated to oral health. Remember that your mouth is a window to the health of your whole body. Be open to your dentist recommending lifestyle changes that will ultimately improve both your oral health and your total body health.

BlabberMouth!

SECTION 13

THE HEALTHY NATION

IN THE PREFACE to **BlabberMouth!**, Dr. Susan talks about her reasons for writing the book—starting with the declining health of her patients and our population as a whole. For her, it was no longer enough to save patients within the four walls of her office. So the goal of this book is to save thousands of Americans and others around the world who are plagued by poor health.

We've spent all of **BlabberMouth!** telling you about the mouth-body connection. And we hope you've learned as much by reading the book as we have by writing it. But there's a bigger picture we need to look at, one we haven't addressed until now: the U.S. healthcare crisis. We're convinced that as the country looks for solutions, dental practices should and will take on much more responsibility. Dentistry has long played a significant role in preventive care for oral health, but now dental teams can also contribute to total health by helping to diagnose and treat disease in the body.

So in this last section, we're going to circle back to the beginning and take a closer look at the downward trend in American health and its devastating social, emotional and economic impact on our country. In 52, Our Sinking Health, we examine why America's health is declining so rapidly. And we look at a slate of candidates to figure out the answer to this question: Who's responsible? We'll tell you. And we'll also tell you how we can turn things around.

Chapter 53, New Solutions, describes the perfect storm of history, technology and policy that's moved dentists to the foreground in the fight against declining health. This will require dentists to move beyond the teeth and gums, and expand their knowledge, so they can step into new roles as diagnosticians and advocates for total health.

In Chapter 54, Help Yourself to Health, we give you the short list of must-dos to improve your health. Must you do them all? Well, not all at once. We suggest you choose one or two of the eight and really get to work. Once you have those down, you can revisit the list and pick again.

Chapter 55, Inspiring Health, explains how you can encourage healthy habits in your family and friends. We'll tell you right here how not to do it: nudge, plead

275

and nag. Dr. Susan, along with every other dentist and hygienist, has already tried those approaches, just to get more people to floss. It doesn't work. So what does work? Letting your family member or friend lead.

We'll also tell you how to help your community and country to health in Chapter 56, Be a BlabberMouth! From what we've seen, the sugar, tobacco and alcohol industries, along with Big Food and Big Pharma, are more focused on profits than on improving our health. And federal, state and local governments tread a wary path between recommendations and regulations, depending on what the health issue is. That leaves it up to you and us to work from the ground up, so we can all lead healthier, happier, sexier lives.

Chapter 52

OUR SINKING HEALTH: WHO'S RESPONSIBLE?

MAYBE THE MOUTH-BODY CONNECTION would be just an interesting aside for your next cocktail party if it weren't for this simple fact: Overall, the health of our country is sinking.

We are among the wealthiest nations on earth, but we're far from being the healthiest. In the 2010 publication *U.S. Health in International Perspective: Shorter Lives, Poorer Health,* the National Research Council and Institute of Medicine compared the United States with other high-income countries—countries we consider our peers, like Canada, Australia and Japan. The study found Americans die sooner and experience more illness than residents of most of our peer countries.

> ## SECRET
>
> **Of the 17 wealthiest countries, the United States ranks last in life expectancy for males and next to last for females. We also have the highest infant mortality rate and poorer health among our children and adolescents. Turning this around will require every American to address root causes and take action.**

For the first time in U.S. history, a generation—the Baby Boomers—is expected to live longer than their children. Our young adults should be the most prolific members of society, but they suffer from higher levels of obesity, chronic illness, sexually transmitted diseases and depression, making them less likely to lead in innovation and productivity.

Dr. Susan has been looking into mouths for 30 years in Smalltown America, doing her very best to help her patients get healthier. The result? In many cases and despite her best efforts, their oral *and* their overall health have continued to deteriorate. From the cradle to the grave, from the rich to the poor, whether we're women or men, the health of too many of our citizens is worsening. And that's even more pronounced among socioeconomically disadvantaged groups.

As a nation, too many of us are overweight and obese, sleep-deprived, sedentary, depressed, addicted and diseased … not to mention cavity-riddled and gum-infected.

> ## Secret
> The number of people afflicted by chronic diseases like heart disease, stroke, cancer, diabetes and respiratory ailments continues to rise—which explains why 75 percent of our nation's healthcare expenditure is for preventable chronic disease. We need to shift our focus from identifying and treating disease to preventing it.

Why are we getting sicker?

Given that we have some of the finest doctors and most advanced medical technology in the world—and that we spend more on medical care per person than just about any other country on earth—why are we not the healthiest nation in the world?

If you read Section 11, The Addicted Nation, you know why. The addictions we discuss there impact the health of our bodies and our mouths. We can sum up those addictions again right now: painkillers and other drugs, alcohol, tobacco, sugar, sweetened beverages, caffeine and processed food. And there's yet another addiction: sitting. Too many people spend too much time on their butts, in vehicles and in front of TVs and computers and gaming consoles.

Finally—though many people don't realize how critical this is—too many Americans don't take proper care of their teeth and gums. We think our dentists can treat gum disease and restore decayed or lost teeth. For the most part, they can; but if you leave the chair and change nothing else, the oral diseases will continue—as will the ill effects on your total health.

Our doctors, no matter how educated and excellent—and they are—cannot solve our health problems. How could they when we get to see them for only 15 minutes? That's enough time to listen to our immediate concerns, examine us quickly, write a costly prescription and speed off to the next patient. Our insurance system rewards efficiency, not results. So doctors have only enough time to solve the issue *du jour*, not to discuss the underlying cause or facilitate a behavior change. This is sick care, not healthcare and, in the long run, it's not helping.

Don't look now!

The impact of poor health on the quantity and quality of American lives is bad enough; but the fiscal impact is like a train wreck waiting to happen. We just can't bear to look.

Adlai Stevenson summed it up nicely: "Man is a strange animal. He generally cannot read the handwriting on the wall until his back is up against it."

We now spend $315 billion annually on cardiovascular disease alone. But thanks to the aging baby boomers, by 2030 the cost is expected to *quadruple* to $1.2 trillion.

In 2012, doctors treated 17 million people for type 2 diabetes at a cost of $245 billion. But by 2050, the Centers for Disease Control and Prevention estimates that as many as one in three Americans will be diabetic—more than 100 million people. Do the math and then ask yourself if we can afford another trillion dollars to treat diabetes?

And these are the price tags for only two diseases.

It's clear that our current approach to health is not working. Maybe that's because we are fighting an uphill battle as our society's lifestyle and values change. Partly it's because the treatments we have been rendering may provide short-term gains but do not change the downward trends.

But who's fault is it?

Is it my fault or your fault for living so haphazardly?

Is it the Food and Drug Administration's fault for not setting and enforcing nutrition goals?

Is it the food industry's fault for letting our commercial food supply become a nutrition-free zone?

Is it the medical community's fault for prescribing a pill for an ill rather than taking the time to develop personalized wellness strategies?

Is it the pharmaceutical industry's fault for spending more on consumer advertising and free samples than on all of research and development?

Is it our legislators' fault for letting the United States be one of two countries worldwide that let drug companies market directly to the consumer?

The answer is *Yes!* six times over, to these questions. We are *all* at fault.

It's time to acknowledge that our current approach to health-ifying our people is broken. But who's responsible for fixing us?

> # Secret
>
> **Health is not just the absence of disease; it's living with energy, vitality, creativity, mental clarity and optimism. That kind of health requires adequate rest, sound nutrition, daily exercise, good oral hygiene and the ability to fend off physical and emotional stress.**

Who's responsible?

Who's responsible? We are. Health must be the responsibility of the individual, his or her family, friends, neighbors, the healthcare community, the government, the entire nation.

It's easy to start with the obvious, and look to the medical or dental community to take charge. But as our country, our world, gets sicker, medical teams get more burned out. Keeping their enthusiasm, hope and intrinsic drive alive is daunting. Clinicians need to keep a constant eye on new evidence, more effective preventive and treatment practices, and be willing to respond. They must also admit to patients when they have been wrong and implement change that improves the outcome for you and your family.

Just as physicians should no longer look right past your mouth to evaluate your throat, dental teams should be able to recognize signs of sickness, screen for them, educate patients and help manage and monitor many diseases that extend beyond the oral cavity. It's the future of both professions—and it's the right thing to do to help restore health in our country.

At the same time, you also need to play a role—to encourage your doctors to bridge the gap between oral medicine and total body medicine, and your dentist to realize the vital role he or she plays in identifying risk factors for disease and promoting healthy behaviors.

Thomas Edison said, "The doctor of the future will give no evidence, but will instruct his patient in the care of the human frame, in diet and in the cause and prevention of disease."

We've been instructed, not just by our doctors but by the government as well, that to prevent chronic disease, we should avoid tobacco, eat nutritious foods, exercise and use alcohol responsibly. Failing to follow these behaviors is associated with 40 percent of deaths in the United States.

So how many of us follow that advice ourselves? And even if we do, that's just a start. If we're going to beat the healthcare crisis and become a healthy nation once again, every one of us must also play an active part in helping our families and friends, our community and country to find health.

Let's get going ...

Quickstart to health

1. Be an advocate for your own health.

Stay up on new developments in medical and dental science. Ask your physician and dentist about new information that could make a difference in your wellness.

2. Recognize the role oral health plays in your total health.

You can't be in optimal overall health if your oral health is compromised. Make sure your physician knows if you're dealing with any oral health issues—and your dentist knows about any systemic diseases you're experiencing.

3. Be aware that many serious chronic diseases are also preventable.

That includes serious oral diseases, including tooth decay and periodontitis, and the Top 5 Killers: heart disease, cancer, stroke, diabetes and respiratory disease. We talk more about these in Section 4, The Oral Accomplice to 5 Chronic Killers.

Chapter 53

NEW SOLUTIONS: DENTISTS' GROWING ROLE

IN THE FEBRUARY 23, 2015, ISSUE of *Time* magazine, the CEO of drugstore giant CVS Health, Larry Merlo, tells the public about the CVS MinuteClinics® you may soon see popping up around the country.

In addition to the vaccinations available at the back of drugstores, you can also get a diagnosis for common illnesses such as strep throat, bladder infections, pink eye and acne. Your prescription is written right there, conveniently enough, a win-win for the drugstore and the pharmaceutical companies.

Who's doing the diagnosis? The CVS MinuteClinic® is staffed by a nurse practitioner or physician assistant, depending on state requirements. They do help make healthcare, or more aptly *sick care*, easier to access and more affordable.

That's good but doesn't go far enough to prevent disease or promote wellness. In fact, it fosters the pill-for-an-ill approach to health. And this approach is being introduced not just at CVS, but also at all the other major drugstore chains, as well as retail establishments with in-house pharmacies.

But there's another option. A perfect storm has brought to the forefront new partners who can help physicians by taking on many of the tasks of preventive care, wellness and health advocacy. These partners are the members of your dental team, of course. Let's take a look at how the pieces have come together to address the healthcare crisis with a new model of care.

Putting the pieces together

A history of preventive care: To some extent, dentistry has been focused on promoting wellness for more than 100 years. For about half the population—who schedule the suggested 6-month preventive appointments with a dental hygienist—the purpose of the visit isn't to treat any particular ailment. As such, these visits mark the most regular *preventive* relationship in healthcare.

Time for dialogue and counseling: One significant advantage to letting dental teams assist in primary healthcare screening and disease prevention is that dental visits take longer than medical appointments do. In most cases, a dental preventive visit lasts 50 to 60 minutes, whereas your typical medical office visit lasts about 15 minutes.

New tools like salivary diagnostics: Dental offices are also being called to the forefront of disease diagnostics. As we discuss in Chapter 50, Salivary Diagnostics, the number of diseases your dental team will be able to screen for quickly and conveniently is growing rapidly. That includes surveys and fingerstick blood tests that can forewarn you of prediabetes and diabetes.

Medical and dental information trends: Trends like electronic medical records and expanded insurance reimbursements will promote the total health cause as well. First, the federal mandate that healthcare providers use electronic records helps everyone—physicians, dentists and others—to collaborate conveniently. Providers can also retrieve accurate, current and complete medical and dental information as well as insurance billing, whether it's for oral or systemic health.

Combined billing and insurance: That brings up another change—a move toward combining both medical and dental insurance under one umbrella. This will make it easier for dental offices to be reimbursed by your medical insurance company for primary diagnostics, such as saliva and/or blood testing for chronic inflammation, diabetes, hypertension, human papillomavirus, human immunodeficiency virus, cortisol stress reactions and nutritional deficiencies. Reimbursement may also cover treatment for snoring and obstructive sleep apnea, temporomandibular joint or facial pain, dietary counseling to alleviate acid reflux and food sensitivities, and coaching for smoking cessation.

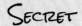

> **S**ECRET
>
> A progressive dentist and hygienist will listen to your health concerns and grow in their understanding of your oral and systemic conditions. They can serve as your advocates and help bridge gaps among your other healthcare providers.

Taking on a new role

The time may be right for dentists to take on a growing and critical role in the healthcare crisis, but they also need to agree to expanded responsibilities. Currently this growing role has been adopted by only 2 percent of the dental profession, according to total health advocates at Henry Schein Corporation, the largest U.S. dental, medical and veterinary equipment, service and business solutions firm. The company is a leader in moving dental practices toward the total health mindset. Still the progress is expected to be slow and steady, according to John Chatham, vice president of Global Sales and Leadership Development.

"Remember, the west was won by pioneers in covered wagons, not jet planes," he recently reminded Dr. Susan. "I expect trends will be very different one year from now and one year after that."

Why is taking on an expanded role so arduous? Change itself is difficult. Human nature often leads us to settle into the comfort of familiarity. That's true even if the entire dental team could find deep intrinsic reward in helping patients create healthy lifestyles.

Transitioning from a traditional to a total health practice means dental teams must learn research-based concepts and change current practices based on that evidence. Dr. Susan can attest to the resources, both in time and money, that must be spent to achieve advanced levels of education in total health, as well as face-to-face facilitation skills.

Success also depends on building collaborative, referral relationships with trusted physicians and other dental practitioners. Once risk factors and systemic disease threats are identified, they can be treated in collaboration with these professionals. Likewise medical teams need to become savvier in identifying health-threatening oral disease and referring patients to the appropriate dentist for attention. In truth, this collaborative approach between dentistry and medicine has not been overly successful in the past. Still Dr. Susan predicts a change in response to the mounting evidence for oral-systemic links and the sophistication dentists are gaining in screening for and diagnosing systemic diseases.

This also means we must continue our shift from the patriarchal medicine model, in which the physician or dentist diagnoses the condition and tells you what to do next, to a facilitated wellness model, where you and your healthcare provider engage in a shared conversation—one that helps you uncover personal solutions to achieve a lifetime of health.

Making the leap

The total health dental practice may not be a fit for everyone. But for those of you who believe you'd benefit from a healthcare team who can track your overall health, identify early signs or risks of both oral and systemic disease, and develop strategies to improve your health, then it's a fit for you.

We already said that only 2 percent of U.S. dental practices operate this way, so finding a total health dental practice is another challenge. Check with your current dental team first—maybe they're moving toward a total health practice. If so, encourage them to read **BlabberMouth!** and share the knowledge you've gained.

If your dental team doesn't plan to expand their scope of practice in this direction, perhaps they can recommend another practice in your community focused on total health. You may also be able to get a recommendation for a total health dentist from a periodontist—a specialist in gum disease with knowledge of the dental community in your area.

No matter where you end up, plan on learning together with your dental team and being patient in the process. Encourage the transition and stay curious about new information. Don't be afraid to ask about the thinking behind recommendations and how it fits with published research. Some dentists learn by reading journals, others by studying with experts in the field, but you don't have to be a research buff yourself to gauge how committed your dental team is to keeping up with advances to provide you with the best care possible.

Quickstart to health

1. Look for a total health dental practice.

Total health practices are the way of the future, but you won't find many yet. Start by having a conversation with your own dental team. Encourage a transformation by talking about what you've learned and asking questions about their plans for the future of the practice.

2. Stay curious about recommendations based on scientific evidence.

Don't be afraid to ask for more detail about what your dental team sees and why they make specific recommendations. With any disease, always ask help in identifying the cause.

3. Be patient as your dental office transitions to a total health practice.

The journey is long and slow, with new knowledge and technology continually changing the path.

Chapter 54

HELP YOURSELF TO HEALTH: EIGHT KEY POINTS

THROUGHOUT **BlabberMouth!**, we've given you lots of history, self-screening tools, a few *Aha* moments and many ways to quickstart your health. At this point, you may be overwhelmed or confused about what to do with all that information. So here we're emphasizing the eight key strategies that Dr. Susan believes are the best ways to improve your overall health.

Everyone's health journey is different, so these are not in priority order. Read through the whole list and check off those you've already tackled. Then choose your next challenge. Set a timeline, build a plan and share it with a trusted accountability partner. Maybe that's your best friend, spouse or even your dental hygienist. When you've accomplished your goal, don't forget to celebrate your success before choosing a new challenge.

1. Cut sugar and increase fiber.

Most health experts now agree that chronic sugar consumption is the primary cause of obesity and leads to obesity-related illness. Chronic sugar intake leads to fat accumulation, fatty liver disease, unhealthy cholesterol ratios, heart disease, type 2 diabetes—and that's just the start of the list. Sugar is also the primary cause of the world's most rampant and preventable dental disease: tooth decay.

Remember that the World Health Organization recommends we cut our sugar consumption down to 5 percent of our daily caloric intake in total. If you're an average-sized person, you probably consume about 2,000 calories a day—so no more than 100 calories should be sugar. That's 26 grams or 6.2 teaspoons a day. If you drink soda, note that you need to limit your consumption to two-thirds of a 12-ounce can—for the entire day. And none of your other food can contain sugar.

To tame your insulin response and reduce the negative impact sugar has on your body, increase your fiber. The Institute of Medicine recommends about 38 grams each day for men and 25 grams a day for women, although many nutritionists suggest we eat much more. For most people, that's about double what we consume. You can meet the fiber goal by eating more fruits, vegetables, nuts, legumes and whole grains. Go online and download a fiber content chart and start keeping a log. You'll be amazed at how much better you feel, even within your first week of upping your fiber.

2. Read the labels on the food you buy and avoid additives that aren't food.

Eating restaurant-prepared meals, fast food and processed or prepackaged foods means you're eating a lot of hidden ingredients. Often these ingredients can put you at risk for obesity and obesity-related diseases, high blood pressure, fatty liver disease, and gut and skin problems. Many of these result in chronic systemic inflammation from a sensitivity to chemically processed, genetically modified or sugar-, salt- or fat-laden food.

If you take a look at the ingredients and don't recognize them as food, there's a reason: They aren't food. That doesn't mean you can never eat processed food again. Our bodies are equipped to clear away some foreign substances—but overload it with too much for too long, and your body will let you know with a negative reaction.

Stick with *whole foods* as much as possible. And if you eat dairy or meat, you want to know that the animal was not munching a bunch of chemicals during its lifetime that are going to end up stored in your body fat.

Dr. Susan's rule on eating processed foods? You can visit there, but you cannot live there. Stay too long and your health will suffer.

3. Break away from addiction.

If you are dependent on anything—sugar, tobacco, alcohol, caffeine, junk food, prescription drugs used for other purposes, marijuana or other street drugs—your health is in jeopardy. Addiction is also psychologically damaging, as you carry it around like a monkey on your back. If you're addicted now or ever have been, you already know that breaking free is not easy; that's how you know it's addiction.

But you can take your first step today. Find help—a program, sponsor or accountability partner. Fixing addiction is never as easy on our own. And it's a one-day-at-a-time job—but remember, days add up to weeks and months and years, until you're living a longer, healthier and happier life.

4. Get moving.

You'll notice there's not a chapter on exercise in **BlabberMouth!** That's not because the authors, both regular exercisers, didn't consider it. But this isn't the mouth's area of expertise; it's the whole body's. We do know that a sedentary lifestyle is associated with weight gain, loss of mental clarity, high blood pressure, heart disease, diabetes, anxiety, depression and even colon cancer.

So we urge you to get at least 30 minutes of exercise at least five days a week. The benefits include helping you to manage your weight, enhance your mood, boost your energy, improve your sleep quality and enrich your sex life.

5. Bust chronic systemic inflammation (CSI).

Inflammation is the body's natural 24/7 defense against injury, and bacterial or viral attack. But when inflammation becomes chronic—meaning it never goes away—it becomes health- and life-threatening. Use the CSI Self-Screen in Chapter 9 to determine if you suffer from it. Work with your healthcare providers to investigate your inflammatory blood markers and to identify the source of your inflammation. Possibilities include gum disease, insulin resistance, lack of sleep, stress, food allergy or sensitivity, chronic obstructive pulmonary disorder or other conditions. Once you've identified a cause, worth with your physician and dentist to eliminate it.

6. Choose a healthcare team committed to helping you achieve your goals.

The quality and quantity of your life are partly in the hands of your healthcare providers. You rely on their philosophies, hunches, tests, diagnoses, recommendations and treatments. That's why it's so critical to find healthcare providers who share your health values, listen to you and collaborate with you and other members of your healthcare team when necessary. Take another look at Chapter 47, The High-Touch Practice, for guidance on choosing a team.

7. Become your own health advocate.

If you're an adult, chances are no one cares about your health as much as you do. Keep track of your medical and dental signs and symptoms, screenings, tests and treatments on a computer or in a notebook. If you suspect a disease or have a diagnosis, do some quality learning on the Web. If you're taking prescription medications, read up on the long-term health risks. Never stop asking questions—even if the questions stay the same, the answers may change as knowledge evolves.

8. Brush and floss, and visit your dentist regularly.

You knew we were going to say this, but that's OK: Great oral health really does help you live longer and better. If you've neglected your home dental care or avoided your dentist for any length of time, start here. Good oral hygiene can make a major difference in your systemic health, but so does the diagnosis of silent diseases, such as decay, periodontal disease, occlusal disease and oral cancer. Keep your mouth healthy by treating any diagnosed decay and gum disease immediately, avoiding chronic exposure to sugar and acidic foods, and cutting out tobacco and excessive alcohol.

Chapter 55

Inspiring Change: Help Your Friends and Family to Health

Do you have a friend or family member whose health habits make you crazy? Of course you do. You want your significant other to quit smoking, your daughter to cut out soda and your best friend to lose weight. You've tried nudging, pleading, even nagging, but none of those have worked.

Dr. Susan can relate—she nudged, pleaded, nagged and flat-out told people to floss for about 15 of her 30 years as a dentist. Did they floss? No. When someone did pick up a flossing habit and she asked why, they almost never said "because you told me to." And that led Dr. Susan to shift from her old teach-and-tell method to the art of facilitation.

Educate versus facilitate

The word *educate* comes from the word *educe*, which means "to bring out." If you've tried to "bring out" a desire in your friend to drop just 10 pounds, you know it's not that simple. But the root of *facilitate* is *facile*, which means "to make a process easy."

Your job is to make change easy for your friend or family member. You do that by helping her get attached to a better outcome and map her own journey to get from here to there.

As one of Susan's favorite authors, Dr. Rachel Naomi Remen, says, "A healer is any person who can see another person's wholeness better than they can at any given moment."

Notice the shift from seeing your friend's brokenness—her sickness—to seeing her wholeness—her wellness. Your friend will be likely to change behavior only if the new behavior supports her new, more desirable picture of herself in that healthier state.

Focus on the future

Let's give you an example. Dr. Susan's friend Anne has diabetes, heart disease and periodontitis. She understands that poor diet, lack of exercise and smoking contribute to her illnesses. And yet she continues to gorge on sugar and fat, rarely takes the stairs (let alone hits the gym) and believes a few cigarettes a day won't harm her.

Anne doesn't want another lecture—she's a sneak eater, a closet smoker and already feels shamed by her doctors. So how can Dr. Susan turn things around?

" SECRET

Lecturing stimulates defensiveness and resistance to change. And it usually keeps your friend's focus on her sickness. Asking good questions and listening with compassion can help shift her focus toward impact— what it would be like to be well. "

The key is to acknowledge the past, recognize the present and then get focused on the future. Here's how: Accept your friend's complaints about the past and how she got to this point. Honor her present conditions, since that's her starting point. And guide her into a vivid description of her desired outcome.

Curiosity is the key. Be an ask-it-all, not a know-it-all. Ask how she would like to feel, to look, to be. Stay curious as long as you can, digging deeper into the possibilities. How would her energy be if she lost 10 pounds? What would change about her life is she could control her diabetes through diet and exercise? How would others experience her differently if she didn't smoke? What would this mean for her personal relationships? What else might she want to accomplish, what could she accomplish, if only she were healthy?

" SECRET

Facilitating health change behavior requires patience. Wait for your friend to get attached to her future vision and describe its possible impact. Then you can begin asking questions about realistic strategies to get from here to there. "

How-to advice will be helpful only once your friend or family member has exhausted her own ideas on making changes. Even then, remember to ask permission to give advice. Finally challenge her to make commitments by speaking them out loud and writing them down. Lifestyle change is usually an evolution, not a revolution, so every baby step is progress.

The accountability partnership

For each of us, keeping a resolution is a challenge. A *Forbes* article published on New Year's Day 2013 revealed that although 40 percent of us make New Year's resolutions, only 8 percent of us achieve them. Dr. Susan finds when her patients make a clear promise to someone else—anyone else—it increases the odds for success. So when a patient states a plan to change a behavior, the dental team likes to collect a "promise card" with a personal commitment written in the patient's own handwriting.

The blank promise cards come from a social movement and non-profit company called **"because I said I would."** Alex Sheen founded the company in tribute to his dad—an ordinary guy who was an extraordinary promise keeper. The company's mission is to strengthen humanity's will by helping hold people accountable to their commitments. If you'd like to learn more, visit www. BecauseIsaidIwould.com.

Your dentist, hygienist, doctor or nurse practitioner can be an accountability partner, and so can you. Ask permission and then establish a comfortable time frame for check-ins with your friends and family members. They may want to touch base every week or two or to talk every day—especially now that you're no longer an irritator but a confidante, encourager, inspirer and healer.

Your steps to better health

1. Recognize that we all have a responsibility to help friends and family improve their health.

Given the healthcare crisis that's confronting America, we all need to be our brother's keeper. Think continued compassionate action.

2. Learn and practice the art of facilitation.

Become the change agent for friends and family members who would benefit from developing new habits.

3. Help loved ones see the future.

Only after your friend or family member gets attached to an outcome and imagines her new self can you help her map a journey to get from here to there.

4. Request permission to give advice.

Be an ask-it-all, not a know-it-all. No one likes to be lectured. Share your ideas only after your friend has exhausted his and you've asked his permission.

5. Ask for commitments out loud and in writing.

People who tell others of their goals and put them down in writing are far more likely to achieve them.

6. Realize that behavior change is an evolution, not a revolution.

Be compassionate and think in baby steps. As your friends and loved ones move the needle toward better health, it will become easier for them to make even more positive changes.

Chapter 56

BE A BLABBERMOUTH! HELP YOUR COMMUNITY AND COUNTRY TO HEALTH

IN OUR SEARCH FOR SOLUTIONS TO THE U.S. and worldwide health crisis, we've called on medical and dental teams to adopt a new model for patient care that ties together oral and overall health. Healthcare providers play a vital role in identifying risk factors for disease and for suggesting lifestyle changes before prescribing drugs.

We've called on you to make changes to improve your own health, whether you're cutting out sugar or starting to exercise. We've even asked you to be your brother's keeper—and your sister's and your best friend's—by inspiring them to make health behavior changes.

And now we want you to take an even bigger step, and become a BlabberMouth! That means you recognize that the United States is facing an unprecedented healthcare crisis—and that we can't look to government or industry for the solution.

The government, whether federal, state or local, walks a cautious line between recommendations and regulations and their financial impact, depending on the threat to health and the economy. As a country, we expect the government to provide health education, whether that's information on the dangers of smoking, changes to the nutrition labeling mandated by the Food and Drug Administration or support for First Lady Michelle Obama's "Let's Move" campaign.

But we balk at regulations, especially when they're targeted at something we enjoy, such as food. We find it much easier to regulate the tobacco industry, with its single product known to cause harm in any amount. But it's not so easy to regulate the food industry, with its multitude of products that may not be harmful in small doses but are potentially disastrous in large doses.

Many of those who could be influential—Big Food, Big Pharma, the sugar, tobacco and alcohol industries—won't be unless a change would also positively impact their profit centers. That will take incentive, creativity and just plain old wanting to do the right thing. But we can also influence these industries, with personal choice on what our hard-earned dollars will support.

In the end, the most powerful motivator for health change may be peer approval. For example, governments regulated drunk driving for years; but after Candice Lightner founded Mothers Against Drunk Driving (MADD), following the death of her 13-year-old daughter in a hit-and-run incident, the peer pressure against driving drunk mounted and deaths from drunk driving began to drop.

Likewise your influence with your peers and in your community can make the biggest impact on our health. There is power in community—in reaching out to neighbors in a grassroots effort to help them learn about America's sinking health and to encourage changes in health behavior. We need to do this before illness cripples our country. We'd like to challenge each of you to start by adopting just one of the 10 actions we list below (or more—we don't want to limit you).

Secret

Don't keep any of **BlabberMouth!** a secret! Sharing evidence-based health information with your friends, family and community makes a positive difference in our country's health.

1. Keep learning. You've read **BlabberMouth!** Now keep reading and learning from research-based sources. But remember that evidence changes as scientists learn more. Always be open to changing your beliefs.

2. Keep asking questions. Dr. Michael Glick, editor of the *Journal of the American Dental Association* and dean of the State University of New York-Buffalo School of Dentistry, recently reminded an audience of professionals, "It's not about what we know. It's about the questions we ask as a result of what we've learned." Asking good questions will help sharpen our focus on better solutions.

3. Start a health blog or a Facebook group. One way to learn more about health issues and to engage in thought-provoking discussions is to share your knowledge. You'll find that health is almost as explosive a subject as politics and religion.

4. Organize a health book club. Read and discuss books that address some of the key issues in health, from Robert Lustig's *Fat Chance: The Bitter Truth about Sugar* to Bale and Doneen's *Beat the Heart Attack Gene* to

5. Organize a health study club. Members could take turns presenting and leading discussions on health information. Also invite health experts to present their thoughts on critical issues in your community.

6. Support nutrition programs in your schools and workplace. Encourage the replacement of junk food and soda in cafeterias and vending machines with healthy options—especially for those learning habits that could last a lifetime.

7. Support physical activity programs in your schools and workplace. Make physical activity a part of life every day. If you're a parent, help out with a school sports program, even if you never played a sport. Encourage your employer to offer on-site exercise, a fitness challenge or recreational sports teams. And advocate for walking paths and bike routes in your community.

8. Support anti-tobacco programs in your schools. Did you know that 90 percent of smokers start tobacco use before they turn 18? Help form school-age children's ideas on smoking before the tobacco industry does.

9. Support programs and policies to reduce alcohol and drug consumption, especially among minors. You don't have to be a parent to recognize the dangers of the underage and binge drinking that runs rampant at schools and colleges. In states where marijuana is legal, the age for first-time users is getting younger. Use of alcohol and drugs damages developing brains. Help kids learn about health and develop good habits that will serve them for a lifetime.

10. Help underserved kids learn to brush and floss. Review Chapter 35, Your Toothbrush and Chapter 37, Your Floss. The gift of your time, along with toothbrushes, toothpaste and floss, could make a significant difference in a child's oral health—one that will lead them to a healthier, happier, sexier life in years to come.

Acknowledgments

Dr. Susan

This book has been inspired and blessed by so many people in my life, not the least of whom are the patients featured in these pages. You have taught me through your trials and then granted me permission to tell others. May the generous gift of your stories come back to you a thousand fold.

Writing this book really began six years ago, when I accepted the challenge to write a monthly article for *Healthy and Fit Magazine*. Sixty-five articles later, a publicist named Bruce Serbin inspired the concept of **BlabberMouth!** Thanks, Bruce.

I am most grateful to my mother and father, both of whom were journalists and writers, among other things. They each infused me with an extraordinary appreciation for the written word and, along with my step-mom ("bonus-mom"), they encouraged me to pursue my dreams to help and to serve … but also to keep writing throughout my life.

Next, I owe a debt of gratitude to my dedicated dental team members. I couldn't have accomplished a total health practice with an ordinary team. Sherry, Georgette, Jean, Kelly, Sally, Corri, Emily, Anna, Molly, and Elizabeth flock, like a band of angels, over our patients. My inspiration grows from watching them move mountains and pave clear paths for people to rediscover what it is to be healthy. Special thanks goes to my personal assistant Molly, who has reviewed **BlabberMouth!** twice over and who continues to encourage its critical place in the health crisis. I'm grateful to our other reviewers too—Bethany, Michael, Steve, Shiraz, KaLee, Meg and Stan.

I extend a special tribute to a few beacons of light among my many treasured teachers: Dr. Peter Dawson, Dr. Bob Frazer, Dr. Rachael Remen, Dr. Frank Spear, Dr. John Kois, Terry Goss, Janis DuPratte, Dr. Wit Wilkerson, Mary Osborn, Dr. Amy Doneen, Dr. Brad Bale, Dr. Lee Ostler, Dr. Michael Glick, Jen McGuire, MaryBeth Palmer-Gierlinger, Dr. Saleh Aldasouqi and my personal miracle-worker, Dr. Roberta Zapp. Without her, center stage in my life 43 years ago, there would be no book.

I also give a heap of gratitude to our *unmentioned* patients, for your dedication and encouragement to our practice transition from a traditional dental practice to a total health dental practice. I appreciate your every raised eyebrow, the telltale sign that a secret has just been received.

Last, but certainly not least, I want to thank my co-author, Diana, a professional writer whose work I have admired for decades. Her wonderful talent, as well as her keen eye on the organization and consistency of **BlabberMouth!**, has certainly raised this work above my already high expectations.—S.S.M.

Diana

Writing this book has been an adventure, complete with quicksand, snake pits and enough summits to make the quest worthwhile. Along the way I've explored new ideas, learned a bit about the world and discovered what I can accomplish when I make a commitment.

But I didn't do it alone. So I want to start by thanking Susan for asking me to write **BlabberMouth!** with her. I admire her creativity, passion and leadership in her profession. The many months of research and writing for **BlabberMouth!** gave me the chance to learn much that will improve my own health and life, and that I can share with family and friends to make theirs better too.

Speaking of family, I want to thank my Mom for her unflagging interest in **BlabberMouth!** The months after my father's passing have been the most difficult of her life, but she never failed to ask how the book was progressing. Thanks also to Gloria and Frank Womble for supporting my writing career. I also find extraordinary inspiration and encouragement from my cousins, particularly Terri Kightlinger Nigro, who generously offered to copy edit the book.

I'm lucky to have the support of many friends as well, especially Anita Grinich, Anne Guest, and Blossom and Troy Savage, who invited my husband and me for dinner and got an unexpected lecture on dental health. Thanks also to the many pals who kindly claimed they couldn't wait to see the book—it's here!

Some friends played a dual role, including Meg Kenagy, my consultant for all things related to writing and style. As a reviewer, she was joined by Dr. Bethany Piziks, Molly Day, KaLee Henderson, Dr. Stan Dorrow, Michael Smallegan and Shiraz Fagan. Your honesty and insight improved every chapter of **BlabberMouth!**

I also want to thank Tracy Walker, who did yeowoman's duty trying to pin down resources for some of our off-the-wall research requests. My longtime colleague Deon Staffelbach showed again why he's one of my fave designers by creating a book cover everyone loves at first sight. Claire Nee, a young dental hygiene student, provided the fun and helpful illustrations sprinkled throughout **BlabberMouth!** And a special debt of gratitude goes to Suzette Perry and Infinity Graphics for putting together a polished book.

A shout-out also to Cody DeCouteau, who curled up all 75 pounds of his furry self to fit under my desk and keep me company while I wrote. Thanks also, Cody, for coming around with a bone or stuffed animal when a break seemed in order.

Above all, I want to thank my husband, Duane DeCouteau. You encouraged me to write this book even though you knew how much more demanding your own life would be as a result. For months, while I wrote and researched and edited, you selflessly supported me so that I could pursue a dream. It's not too much to say that **BlabberMouth!** wouldn't exist without your love and support. You're my hero.—D.K.D.

Blabber Mouth!

BIOS

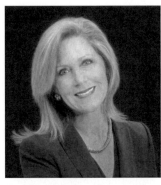

Dr. Susan

Dr. Susan Maples is a national thought leader in oral-systemic health. She is the originator of the *Hands-On Learning Lab*™, a self-care total-health science curriculum for children age 2 to 18, and SelfScreen.net, a series of health assessment screening tools for adults. She has led a dental practice in Holt, Michigan, for 30 years.

Dr. Susan recently partnered with Dr. Saleh Aldasouqi, chairman of Michigan State University's Department of Endocriniology, to develop a dental office screening tool for diabetes and prediabetes. The study earned first place recognition at the 2015 meeting of the American Association of Clinical Endocrinologists.

In 2012, Susan was named as one of the Top 25 Women in Dentistry (Dentistry Today, September 2012) and the Top 8 Innovators (Incisal Edge magazine, Summer 2012) in Dentistry. In 2013, she was chosen to represent the dentist of the future in the state of Washington.

In addition to her other speaking engagements, Susan currently leads the Total Health and Practice Profitability program for Henry Schein Dental Corporation throughout the United States.

As an entertaining speaker for corporate wellness gatherings, civic organizations, dental teams, medical teams, and study clubs throughout the world, Susan's personal mission is *to positively impact the health of America, by inspiring brave behavior changes among her audience members.* For more information visit DrSusanMaplesSpeaker.com.

Susan holds a bachelor's degree from Denison University, a doctor of dental surgery degree from University of Michigan and a master's degree in business from Madonna University.

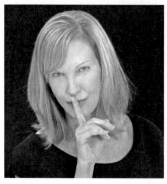

Diana

Diana Kightlinger DeCouteau, is a journalist, essayist, scientist and now author. For more than 25 years, she's worked as a marketing communication specialist for some of the top companies in the world, including General Motors, Hewlett-Packard, Xerox, Visa, Samsung and Intel. Her specialty? Explaining complex concepts in words with no more than three syllables.

For fun, Diana writes articles and essays for everyone from the *Chicago Tribune*, *Washington Post* and *Detroit Monthly* to *Backpacker*, *Discovery* and the New York Academy of Sciences.

Diana is currently exploring her feelings about running (*Will I ever fall in love with dragging my body down the road?*) and recently completed her first marathon. She's now training to qualify for Boston. Read more in her next book, *The Last Best Runner.*

Diana earned a bachelor's degree in geology from University of Maryland and master's degrees in journalism from Michigan State and environmental science from Portland State University. She is a member of Kappa Tau Alpha Journalism Honor Society.

References

Chapter 2

Cephas, K.D., Kim, J., Mathai, R.A., et al. (2011). Comparative analysis of salivary bacterial microbiome diversity in edentulous infants and their mothers or primary caregivers using pyrosequencing. *PLOS One, 6, 323503.*

Dewhirst, F.E., Chen T., Izard J., et al. (2010). The human oral microbiome. *Journal of Bacteriology, 192,* 5002-17.

Loesche, Walter. (1987). *Caries: A Treatable Infection.* Ann Arbor, Michigan: University of Michigan School of Dentistry.

National Children's Oral Health Foundation. (2015). Facts about tooth decay. Retrieved from http://www.ncohf.org/resources/tooth-decay-facts.

Templeton, S. (2014, July 13). Rotten teeth put 26,000 children in hospital. *The Sunday Times* (London, U.K.).

Chapter 4

Eke, P.I., Dye, B.A., Wei, L., et al. (2012). Prevalence of periodontitis in adults in the United States: 2009 and 2010. *Journal of Dental Research, 91*(10), 914-20.

Kassebaum, N.J., Bernabé, E., Dahiya, M., et al. (2014). Global burden of severe periodontitis in 1990-2010: A systematic review and meta-regression. *Journal of Dental Research, 93*(11), 1045-53.

Chapter 5

Centers for Disease Control and Prevention. (2005). Trends in oral health status— United States 1988-1994 and 1999-2004. *Morbidity and Mortality Weekly Report, 54,* 1-44.

Centers for Disease Control and Prevention. (2015). Hygiene-related diseases. Retrieved from http://www.cdc.gov/healthywater/hygiene/disease/dental_caries.html.

National Institutes of Health. (2015). Dental caries (tooth decay) in adults (age 20 to 64). Retrieved from http://www.nidcr.nih.gov/DataStatistics/FindDataByTopic/DentalCaries/DentalCariesAdults20to64.htm.

U.S. Department of Health and Human Services, National Institute of Dental and Craniofacial Research, U.S. Public Health Service. (2000). *Oral health in America: Report of the U.S. Surgeon General.* NIH publication no. 00-213. Washington, DC: DHHS, NIDCR, USPHS.

Chapter 8

Centers for Disease Control and Prevention. (2011). Oral health: Preventing cavities, gum disease, tooth loss and oral cancers, at a glance 2011. Retrieved from http://www.cdc.gov/chronicdisease/resources/publications/aag/doh.htm.

World Health Organization. (2012). Oral health fact sheet No. 318, April 2012. Retrieved from http://www.who.int/mediacentre/factsheets/fs318/en/.

Chapter 9

Bale, B., & Doneen, A. (2014). *Beat the heart attack gene: The revolutionary plan to prevent heart disease, stroke, and diabetes.* Wiley: New York, NY.

Johannsen, N.M., Priest, E.L., Dixit, V.D., et al. (2010). Association of white blood cell subfraction concentration with fitness and fatness. *British Journal of Sports Medicine, 44,* 588-93.

Loe, H., Theilade, E., & Jensen, S.B. (1965). Experimental gingivitis in man. *Journal of Periodontology, 36,* 177-87.

Chapter 10

Borgnakke, W.S. (2014). The traveling oral microbiome. In M. Glick (Ed.) *The oral-systemic health connection.* Chicago: Quintessence Publishing Company.

Han, Y.W., Fardini, Y., Chen, C., et al. (2010). Term stillbirth caused by oral *Fusobacterium nucleatum. Obstetrics & Gynecology, 115*(2 Pt 2), 442-5.

Koren, O., Spor A., Felin, J., et al. (2011). Human oral, gut, and plaque microbiota in patients with atherosclerosis. *Proceedings of the National Academy of Sciences of the United States of America, 108,* 4592-8.

Section 4

Centers for Disease Control and Prevention. (2015). Death and mortality. National Center for Health Statistics FastStats website. Retrieved from http://www.cdc.gov/nchs/fastats/deaths.htm.

Editorial. (2009). Tackling the burden of chronic diseases in the USA. *Lancet, 373*(9659), 185. Retrieved from http://www.thelancet.com/journals/lancet/article/PIIS0140-6736(09)60048-9/fulltext.

National Center for Chronic Disease Prevention and Health Promotion. (2009). *The power of prevention: Chronic disease ... The public health challenge of the 21st century.* Retrieved from http://www.cdc.gov/chronicdisease/pdf/2009-Power-of-Prevention.pdf.

Chapter 11

Bale, B., & Doneen, A. (2014). *Beat the heart attack gene: The revolutionary plan to prevent heart disease, stroke, and diabetes.* Wiley: New York, NY.

Friedewald, V.E., Kornman, K.S., Beck, J.D., et al. (2009). The American Journal of Cardiology and Journal of Periodontology Editors' Consensus: Periodontitis and atherosclerotic cardiovascular disease. *American Journal of Cardiology, 104*(1), 59-68.

Pessi, T., Karhunen, V., Karjalainen, P.P., et al. (2013). Bacterial signatures in thrombus aspirates of patients with myocardial infarction. *Circulation, 127*(11), 1219-28.

Chapter 12

American Cancer Society. (2015). Cancer facts & figures 2015. Atlanta, Georgia: American Cancer Society.

Hujoel, P.P., Drangsholt, M. Spiekerman, C., & Weiss, N.S. (2003, May). An exploration of the periodontitis-cancer association. *Annals of Epidemiology, 13*(5), 312-6.

Michaud, D.S., Joshipura, K., Giovannucci, E., & Fuchs, C.S. (2007). A prospective study of periodontal disease and pancreatic cancer in U.S. male health professionals. *Journal of the National Cancer Institute, 99*(2), 171-5.

Michaud, D.S., Liu, Y., Meyer, M., et al. (2008). Periodontal disease, tooth loss and cancer risk in a prospective study of male health professionals. *Lancet Oncology, June 9*(6), 550-8.

Michaud, D.S., Izard, J., Wilhem-Benartzi, C.S., et al. (2013). Plasma antibodies to oral bacteria and risk of pancreatic cancer in a large European prospective cohort study. *Gut, 62*(12), 1764-70.

Shamami, M.S., Shamami, M.S., & Amini, S. (2011). Periodontal disease and tooth loss as risks for cancer: A systematic review of the literature. *Iranian Journal of Cancer Prevention, 4*, 189–98.

Steward, B.W., & Wild, C.P. (Eds.) (2014). *World cancer report 2014.* International Association for Research on Cancer. Geneva: WHO Press.

Tezal, M., Sullivan, M.A., Reid, M.E., et al. (2007). Chronic periodontitis and the risk of tongue cancer. 2007. *Archives of Otoloaryngology—Head and Neck Surgery, 133*(5), 450-4.

Tu, Y-K., Galobardes, B., Smith, G. D., et al. (2007). Associations between tooth loss and mortality patterns in the Glasgow alumni cohort. *Heart, 93*, 1098-1103.

Wynder, E.L., & Bross, I.J. (1957, 18 May). Aetiological factors in mouth cancer: An approach to its prevention. *British Medical Journal.*

References 305

Chapter 13

American Heart Association. (2013). Heart disease and stroke statistics—2013 update: A report from the American Heart Association. *Circulation, 127*, e6-e245.

Joshipura, K.J., Hung, H.C., Rimm, E.B., et al. (2003). Periodontal disease, tooth loss, and incidence of ischemic stroke. *Stroke, 34*, 47-52.

Sfyroeras, G.S., Roussas, N., Saleptsis, V.G., et al. (2012). Association between periodontal disease and stroke. *Journal of Vascular Surgery, 55*(4), 1178-84.

Syrjanen, J., Valtonen, V.S., Iivanainen, M., et al. (1986). Association between cerebral infarction and increased serum bacterial antibody levels in young adults. *Acta Neurologica Scandinavica, 73*(3), 273-8.

World Health Organization. (2010). *Global status report on noncommunicable diseases.* Geneva: World Health Organization.

Wu, T., Trevisan, M., Genco, R.J., et al. (2000). Periodontal disease and risk of cerebrovascular disease: The first national health and nutrition examination survey and its follow-up study. *Archives of Internal Medicine, 160*, 2749-55.

Chapter 14

Aldasouqi, S., & Gossain, V. (2012). Updates on diabetes diagnosis: A historical review of the dilemma of the diagnostic utility of glycohemoglobin A1c and a proposal of a combined glucose-A1c diagnostic method. *Annals of Saudi Medicine, 32*(3), 229-35.

American Diabetes Association (ADA). (2014, May 8). Fast facts: Data and statistics about diabetes. Retrieved from www.diabetes.org.

Centers for Disease Control and Prevention. (2014, August 10). Fast facts on diabetes-2014. Retrieved from http://www.cdc.gov/diabetes/pubs/statsreport14.htm.

Demmer, R.T., Holtfreter, B., Desvarieux, M., et al. (2012). The influence of type 1 and type 2 diabetes on periodontal disease progression: Prospective results from the Study of Health in Pomerania (SHIP). *Diabetes Care, 35*(10), 2036-42.

Graves, D.T., & Kayal, R.A. (2008). Diabetic complications and dysregulated innate immunity. *Frontiers in Biosciences, 13*, 1227-39.

Grossi, S., & Genco, R. (1998). Periodontal disease and diabetes mellitus: A two-way relationship. *Annals of Periodontology, 3*, 51-61.

Herman, W. (2013). The economic costs of diabetes: Is it time for a new treatment paradigm? *Diabetes Care, 36*, 775-6.

Javed, F., Al-Askar, M., Al-Rasheed, A., et al. (2011). Comparison of self-perceived oral health, periodontal inflammatory conditions and socioeconomic status in individuals with and without prediabetes. *American Journal of the Medical Sciences, 344*(2), 100-4.

Noble, D., Mathur, R., Dent, T., et al. (2011). Risk models and scores for type 2 diabetes: Systematic review. *British Medical Journal, 343*, d7163.

Phillips, L., Ratner, R., Buse, J., & Kahn, S. (2014). We can change the natural history of type 2 diabetes. *Diabetes Care, 37*, 2668-75.

Taylor, G. (2001). Bidirectional interrelationship between diabetes and periodontal diseases: An epidemiologic perspective. *Annals of Periodontology, 6*, 99-112.

Taylor, G.W., Burt, B.A., Becker, M.P., et al. (1996). Severe periodontitis and risk for poor glycemic control in subjects with non-insulin-dependent diabetes mellitus. *Journal of Periodontology, 67* (suppl), 1085-93.

Teeuw, W.J., Gerdes, V.E., & Loos, B.G. (2010). Effect of periodontal treatment on glycemic control of diabetic patients: A systematic review and meta-analysis. *Diabetes Care 33*(2), 421-427.

Chapter 15

Centers for Disease Control and Prevention. (2011). National Center for Health Statistics. National health interview survey raw data, 2011. Analysis performed by the American Lung Association Research and Health Education Division using SPSS and SUDAAN software.

Murphy, S.L., Xu, J., & Kochanek, K.D. (2013, May). Centers for Disease Control and Prevention, National Center for Health Statistics. Deaths: Final data for 2010. *National Vital Statistics Reports, 61*(4).

Didilescu, A.C., Skaug, N., Marca, C., et al. (2005). Respiratory pathogens in dental plaque of hospitalized patients with chronic lung disease. *Clinical Oral Investigations, 9*, 141-7.

Hayes, C., Sparrow, D., Cohen, M., et al. (1998). The association between alveolar bone loss and pulmonary function: The VA dental longitudinal study. *Annals of Periodontology, 3*(1), 257-61.

Lopez, A.D., Mathers, C.D., Ezzati, M., et al. (2006). Global and regional burden of disease and risk factors, 2001: Systematic analysis of population health data. *Lancet, 367*, 1747-57.

Scannapieco, F.A., Papandonatos, G.D., & Dunford, R.G. (1998). Associations between oral conditions and respiratory disease in a national sample survey population. *Annals of Periodontology, 3*(1), 251-6.

Scannapieco, F.A., & Ho, A.W. (2001). Potential associations between chronic respiratory disease and periodontal disease: Analysis of National Health and Nutrition Examination Survey III. *Journal of Periodontology, 72*(1), 50-6.

Sharma, N., & Shamsuddin, H. (2011). Association between respiratory disease in hospitalized patients and periodontal disease: A cross-sectional study. *Journal of Periodontology, 82*, 1155-60.

Chapter 16

Dahiya, P. Kamal., R., & Gupta, R. (2012). Obesity, periodontal and general health: Relationship and management. *Indian Journal of Endocrinology Metabolism, 18*(1), 88-93.

Dalla Vecchia, C.F., Susin, C., Rösing, C.K., et al. (2005). Over weight and obesity as a risk indicator for periodontitis in adults. *Journal of Periodontology, 76,* 1721-8.

Deng, T., Lyon, C.J., Minze, L.J., et al. Class II major histocompatibility complex plays an essential role in obesity-induced adipose inflammation. *Cell Metabolism, 17*(3), 411-22.

Greenberg, A.S., & Obin, M.S. (2006). Obesity and the role of adipose tissue in inflammation and metabolism. *American Journal of Clinical Nutrition, 83*(2), 461S-465S.

Khader, U.S., Bawadi, H.A., Haroun, T.F., et al. (2009). The association between periodontal disease and obesity among adults in Jordan. *Journal of Clinical Periodontology, 36,* 18–24.

Olshansky S.J., Passaro, D.J., Hershow, R.C., et al. (2006). A potential decline in life expectancy in the United States in 21st century. *New England Journal of Medicine, 352*(11), 1138-45.

Sarlati, F., Akhondi, N., Ettehad, T., et al. (2008). Relationship between obesity and periodontal status in sample of young Iranian adults. *International Dental Journal, 58,* 36-40.

Stillwell, K.D. Obesity complicates dental health—be proactive! (2015, March 18). Obesity Action Coalition. Retrieved from http://www.obesityaction.org/educational-resources/resource-articles-2/obesity-related-diseases/obesity-complicates-dental-health.

World Health Organization. (2015, January 3). Fact sheet: Obesity and overweight. Retrieved from www.who.int/dietphysicalactivity/publications/facts/obesity/en/.

Ogden, C.L., Carroll, M.D., Kit, B.K., & Flegal, K.M. (2014). Prevalence of childhood and adult obesity in the United States, 2011-2012. *Journal of the American Medical Association, 311*(8), 806-14.

Finkelstein, E.A., Trogdon, J.G., Cohen, J.W., & Dietz, W. (2009). Annual medical spending attributable to obesity: Payer- and service-specific estimates. *Health Affairs, 28*(5), w822-31.

Chapter 17

Han, Y.W., Fardini, Y., Chen, C., et al. (2010). Term stillbirth caused by oral *Fusobacterium nucleatum*. *Obstetrics & Gynecology, 115*(2 Pt 2), 442-5.

Arafat, A.H. (1974). Periodontal status during pregnancy. *Journal of Periodontology, 45,* 641–3.

March of Dimes, PMNCH, Save the Children, WHO. (2012). *Born too soon: The global action report on preterm birth.* Retrieved from http://www.marchofdimes.org/materials/born-too-soon-the-global-action-report-on-preterm-birth.pdf.

Liu, L., Johnson, H.L., Cousens, S., et al. (2012). Global, regional, and national causes of child mortality: An updated systematic analysis for 2010 with time trends since 2000. *Lancet, 379,* 2151-61.

Martin, J.A., Hamilton, B.E., Sutton, P.D., et al. (2009). Births: Final data for 2006. *National Vital Statistics Report, 57,* 1-102.

Pitiphat, W., Gillman, M.S., Joshipura, K.J., et al. (2005). Plasma C-reactive protein in early pregnancy and preterm delivery. *American Journal of Epidemiology, 162,* 1108-13.

Han, Y.W., & Wang, X. (2013). Mobile microbiome: Oral bacteria in extra-oral infections and inflammation. *Journal of Dental Research, 92*(6), 485-91.

Madianos, P.N., Bobetsis, Y.A., & Offenbacher, S. (2013). Adverse pregnancy outcomes (APOs) and periodontal disease: Pathogenic mechanisms. *Journal of Periodontology, 84*(4 supplement), S170-S180.

Han, Y.W., Ikegami, A., & Bissada, N.F. (2006). Transmission of an uncultivated Bergeyella strain from the oral cavity to amniotic fluid in a case of preterm birth. *Journal of Clinical Microbiology, 44,* 1475-83.

Offenbacher, S., Katz, V., Fertik, G., et al. (1996). Periodontal infection as a possible risk factor for preterm low birth weight. *Journal of Periodontology, 67*(10 suppl), 1103-13.

Ide, M., & Papapanou, P.N. Epidemiology of association between maternal periodontal disease and adverse pregnancy outcomes—systematic review. *Journal of Clinical Periodontology, 40*(suppl 14), S181-94.

Chapter 18

Jämsen, E., Varonen, M., Huhtala, H., et al. (2010). Incidence of prosthetic joint infections after primary knee arthroplasty. *Journal of Arthroplasty, 25*(1), 87-92.

Iorio, R., Williams, K.M., Marcantonio, A.J., et al. (2012). Diabetes mellitus, hemoglobin A1C, and the incidence of total joint arthroplasty infection. *Journal of Arthroplasty, 27*(5), 726-9.e1.

Jevsever, D.S., & Abt, E. (2013). The new AAOS-ADA clinical practice guideline on prevention of orthopedic implant infection in patients undergoing dental procedures. *Journal of the American Academy of Orthopedic Surgeons, 21,* 195-197.

Trampuz, A., & Zimmerli, W. (2005). Prosthetic joint infections: Update in diagnosis and treatment. *Swiss Medical Weekly, 135,* 243-51.

Chapter 19

National Highway Traffic Safety Administration. NCSDR/NHTSA Expert Panel on Driver Fatigue and Sleepiness. Drowsy driving and automobile crashes. Retrieved from http://www.nhtsa.gov/people/injury/drowsy_driving1/Drowsy.html.

Harsch, I.A., Konturek, P.C., Koebnick, C., et al. (2003, August). Leptin and ghrelin levels in patients with obstructive sleep apnoea: Effect of CPAP treatment. *European Respiratory Journal, 22*(2), 251-7.

Chapter 20

Koufman, J., Stern, J. & Bauer, M. (2010). *Dropping acid: The reflux diet cookbook & cure.* New York: Reflux Cookbooks.

Lagergren, J., Bergstrom, R., Lindgren, A., & Nyren, O. (1999). Symptomatic gastroesophageal reflux as a risk factor for esophageal adenocarcinoma. *New England Journal of Medicine, 340,* 825–31.

National Cancer Institute. Surveillance, Epidemiology, and End Results Program. SEER STAT fact sheets: Esophageal cancer. Retrieved from http://seer.cancer.gov/statfacts/html/esoph.html.

Ness-Jensen, E., Lindam, A., Lagergren, J., & Hveem, K. (2012). Changes in prevalence, incidence and spontaneous loss of gastro-oesophageal reflux symptoms: A prospective population-based cohort study, the HUNT study. *Gut, 61*(10), 1390-7.

Jacobson, B.C., Somers, S.C., Fuchs, C.F., et al. (2006). Body-mass index and symptoms of gastroesophageal reflux in women. *New England Journal of Medicine, 354,* 2340-8.

Chapter 22

Milgrom P., Weinstein P., & Getz, T. (1995). *Treating fearful dental patients: A patient management handbook* (2nd ed.). Seattle, Wash.: University of Washington, Continuing Dental Education.

Gatchel, R.J., Ingersoll, B.D., Bowman, L., et al. (1983). The prevalence of dental fear and avoidance: A recent survey study. *Journal of the American Dental Association. 107*(4), 609-10.

Chapter 23

Strack, F., Martin, L.L., & Stepper, S. (1988). Inhibiting and facilitating conditions of a human smile: A nonobtrusive test of the facial feedback hypothesis. *Journal of Personality and Social Psychology, 54*(5), 768.

Stevenson, S. (2012, June 25). There's magic in your smile. Guest blog post published by R.E. Riggio. *Psychology Today.* Retrieved from https://www.psychologytoday.com/blog/cutting-edge-leadership/201206/there-s-magic-in-your-smile.

Hyde, S., Satariano, W.A., & Weintraub, J.A. (2006). Welfare dental intervention improves employment and quality of life. *Journal of Dental Research, 85*(1), 79-84.

Duhigg, C. (2012). *The power of habit: Why we do what we do in life and business.* New York: Random House.

Chapter 24

Kessler, R.C., Chiu, W.T., Demler, O., et al. (2005). Prevalence, severity, and comorbidity of 12-month DSM-IV disorders in the National Comorbidity Survey Replication. *Archives of General Psychiatry, 62*(6), 617-27.

Weissman, M.M., Bland, R.C., Canino, G.J., et al. (1996). Cross-national epidemiology of major depression and bipolar disorder. *Journal of the American Medical Association, 276,* 293-9.

O'Neil, A., Berk, M., Veugopal, K., et al. (2014). The association between poor dental health and depression: Findings from a large-scale, population-based study (the NHANES study). *General Hospital Psychiatry, 36*(3), 266-70.

International & American Associations for Dental Research. (2014, March 20). Study links tooth loss to depression and anxiety. [Press release]. Retrieved from http://www.eurekalert.org/pub_releases/2014-03/iaa-slt032014.php.

Section 8 Introduction

Gillison, M., Broutian, T., Pickard R., et al. (2012). Prevalence of oral HPV infection in the United States. *Journal of the American Medical Association, 307*(7), 693-703.

Chapter 27

American Cancer Society. (2014). *Cancer facts & figures 2014.* Atlanta: American Cancer Society.

D'Souza, G., Kreimer, A.R., Viscidi, R. et al. (2007). Case-control study of human papillomavirus and oropharyngeal cancer. *New England Journal of Medicine, 356,* 1944-56.

Fakhry, C., Gillison, M.L., & D'Souza, G. (2014). Tobacco use and oral HPV-16 infection. *Journal of the American Medical Association, 312*(14), 1465-7.

Kaminagakura, E., Villa, L.L., Andreoli, M.A., et al. (2012). High-risk human papillomavirus in oral squamous cell carcinoma of young patients. *International Journal of Cancer, 130*(3), 1726-32.

Laco, J., Vosmikova, H., Novakova, V., et al. (2011). The role of high-risk human papillomavirus infection in oral and oropharyngeal squamous cell carcinoma in non-smoking and non-drinking patients: A clinicopathological and molecular study of 46 cases. *Virchows Archiv, 458*(2), 179-187.

Marur, S., D'Souza, G., Westra, W., et al. (2010). HPV-associated head and neck cancer: A virus-related cancer epidemic. *Lancet Oncology, 11*(8), 781-9.

Mouth Cancer Foundation. (2015, February 9). HPV risks: Mouth cancer and the human papillomavirus. Retrieved from http://www.mouthcancerfoundation.org/patients-guide/hpv-risks.

Schabath, M.B., Thompson, Z.J., Egan, K.M., et al. (2015). Alcohol consumption and prevalence of human papillomavirus (HPV) infection among U.S. men in the HPV in men (HIM) study. *Sexually Transmitted Infections, 91*(1), 61-7.

Chapter 28

Oğuz, F., Eltas, A., Beytur, A., et al. (2013). Is there a relationship between chronic periodontitis and erectile dysfunction? *The Journal of Sexual Medicine, 10*(3), 838-43.

Furuta, M., Ekuni, D., Irie, K., et al. (2011). Sex differences in gingivitis relate to interaction of oral health behaviors in young people. *Journal of Periodontology, 82*(4), 558-65.

Eke, P.I., Dye, B.A., Wei, L., et al. (2012). Prevalence of periodontitis in adults in the United States: 2009 and 2010. *Journal of Dental Research, 91*(10), 914-20.

Chapter 29

Skin Cancer Foundation. (2015, February 10). Squamous Cell Carcinoma (SCC). Retrieved from http://www.skincancer.org/skin-cancer-information/squamous-cell-carcinoma.

Chapter 30

Block, E. (2010). *Garlic and other alliums: The lore and science.* London: Royal Society of Chemistry.

Chapter 32

American Academy of Dental Sleep Medicine. (2015, February 12). Snoring. Retrieved fromhttp://www.aadsm.org/snoring.aspx.

Beninati, W., Harris, C.D., Herold, D.L., et al. (1999). The effect of snoring and obstructive sleep apnea on the sleep quality of bed partners. *Mayo Clinic Proceedings, 74*(10), 955-8.

Chalabi, M. (2014, July 25). Five Thirty Eight, DataLab. Dear Mona, how many couples sleep in separate beds? Retrieved from http://loglr.com/i/102581.

Sardesai, M.G., Tan, A.K., & Fitzpatrick, M. (2003). Noise-induced hearing loss in snorers and their bed partners. *Journal of Otylaryngology, 32*(3), 141-5.

Chapter 35

Klukowska, M., Grender, J.M., & Timm, H. (2012). A single-brushing study to compare plaque removal efficacy of a new power brush to an ADA reference manual toothbrush. *American Journal of Dentistry, 25* Spec. No. A(A), 10A-13A.

Taschner, M., Rumi, K., Master, A.S., et al. (2012). Comparing efficacy of plaque removal using professionally applied manual and power toothbrushes in 4- to 7-year-old children. *Pediatric Dentistry, 34*(1), 61-5.

Chapter 36

Duhigg, C. (2012). *The power of habit: Why we do what we do in life and business.* New York: Random House.

Chapter 37

DeGeneres, E. (2004). *The funny thing is.* New York: Simon & Schuster.

Roizen, M.F. (1999). *Realage: Are you as young as you can be?* New York: Cliff Street Books—HarperCollins Publishers.

Chapter 39

Horowitz, H.S. (1996). The effectiveness of community water fluoridation in the United States. *Journal of Public Health Dentistry, 56*(5 Spec No), 253-8.

Jeevarathan, J., Deepti, A., Muthu, M.S., et al. (2007). Effect of fluoride varnish on *streptococcus mutans* counts in plaque of caries-free children using Dentocult SM strip mutans test: A randomized controlled triple blind study. *Journal of Indian Society* of Pedodontics and Preventive Dentistry, 25(4), 157-63.

National Institute of Dental and Craniofacial Research. (2008, December 20). The story of fluoridation. Retrieved from http://www.nidcr.nih.gov/oralhealth/Topics/Fluoride/TheStoryofFluoridation.htm.

Weintraub, J.A., Ramos-Gomez, F., Jue, B., et al. (2006). Fluoride varnish efficacy in preventing early childhood caries. *Journal of Dental Research, 85*(2), 172-6.

Chapter 40

Centers for Disease Control and Prevention. (2015). National Vital Statistics System mortality data. Retrieved from http://www.cdc.gov/nchs/deaths.htm.

National Institutes of Health. (2011, October). National Institute on Drug Abuse, Research Report Series. *Prescription drugs: Abuse and addiction.* NIH Publication Number 11-4881.

Chapter 41

Blot, W.J., McLaughlin, J.K., Winn, D.M., et al. (1988). Smoking and drinking in relation to oral and pharyngeal cancer. *Cancer Research, 48*, 3282-7.

National Institutes of Health. NIH fact sheet. Oral cancer. Retrieved from http://report. nih.gov/nihfactsheets/ViewFactSheet.aspx?csid=106.

National Institute of Health. Medline Plus. (2015, May 6). Alcoholism and alcohol abuse. Retrieved from http://www.nlm.nih.gov/medlineplus/alcoholism.html.

Chapter 42

American Cancer Society. Guide to quitting smoking. (2014, February 6). Retrieved from http://www.cancer.org/acs/groups/cid/documents/webcontent/002971-pdf.pdf.

International Agency for Research on Cancer. (2007). Smokeless tobacco and some tobacco-specific N-nitrosamines. *IARC Monographs on the Evaluation of Carcinogenic Risks to Humans, 89*. Lyon, France: World Health Organization International Agency for Research on Cancer.

National Institute of Dental and Craniofacial Research. (2012, August). Smokeless tobacco: A guide for quitting. Retrieved from http://www.nidcr.nih.gov/OralHealth/ Topics/SmokelessTobacco/SmokelessTobaccoAGuideforQuitting.htm.

Piano, M.R., Benowitz, N.L., Fitzgerald, G.A., et al. (2010). Impact of smokeless tobacco products on cardiovascular disease: Implications for policy, prevention, and treatment: A policy statement from the American Heart Association. *Circulation, 122*(15), 1520-44.

U.S. Department of Health and Human Services. (2014). *The health consequences of smoking—50 years of progress: A report of the Surgeon General.* Atlanta, GA: U.S. Department of Health and Human Services, Centers for Disease Control and Prevention, National Center for Chronic Disease Prevention and Health Promotion, Office on Smoking and Health.

Chapter 43

Bocarsly, M.E., Powell, E.S., Avena, N.M., & Hoebel, B.G. (2010). High-fructose corn syrup causes characteristics of obesity in rats: Increased body weight, body fat and triglyceride levels. *Pharmacology, Biochemistry and Behavior, 97*(1), 101-06.

Johnson, R.K., Appel, L.J., Brands, M., et al. (2009). Dietary sugars intake and cardiovascular health: A scientific statement from the American Heart Association. *Circulation, 120*, 1011-20.

Hugentobler, S., Ruff., J., Potts, W., et al. (in press). (2015). Compared to sucrose, previous consumption of fructose and glucose monosaccharides reduces survival and fitness of female mice. *The Journal of Nutrition.*

United States Department of Agriculture, Economic Research Service. (2015, April 21). USDA sugar supply: Tables 51-53. U.S. consumption of caloric sweeteners. Retrieved from http://www.ers.usda.gov/data-products/sugar-and-sweeteners-yearbook-tables.aspx.

World Health Organization. (2014, March 5). WHO opens public consultation on draft sugars guidelines. [Press release]. Retrieved from http://www.who.int/mediacentre/news/notes/2014/consultation-sugar-guideline/en/.

Chapter 44

American College of Sports Medicine. (2007). Exercise and fluid replacement position stand. *Medicine and Science in Sports and Exercise, 39*, 377-90.

De Koning, L., Malik, V.S., Kellogg, M.D., et al. (2012). Sweetened beverage consumption, incident coronary heart disease, and biomarkers of risk in men. *Circulation, 125*(14), 1735-41.

Gardner, H., Rundek, T., Market, M., et al. (2012). Diet soft drink consumption is associated with an increased risk of vascular events in the Northern Manhattan Study. *Journal of General Internal Medicine, 27*(9), 1120-6.

Moss, M. (2013). *Salt sugar fat: How the food giants hooked us.* New York: Random House Trade Paperbacks.

Muraki, I., Imamura, F., Manson, J.E., et al. (2013). Fruit consumption and risk of type 2 diabetes: Results from three prospective longitudinal cohort studies. *British Medical Journal, 347*, f5001.

Chapter 45

American Chemical Society. (2005, August 28). Coffee is number one source of antioxidants. *EurekAlert!*. Retrieved from http://www.eurekalert.org/pub_releases/2005-08/acs-cin081905.php.

Hutchison, A. (2011). *Which comes first, cardio or weights?* New York: HarperCollins Publishers.

Lopez-Garcia, E., van Dam, R.M., Li, T.Y., et al. (2008). The relationship of coffee consumption with mortality. *Annals of Internal Medicine, 148*, 904-14.

Substance Abuse and Mental Health Services Association. (2014, 13 March). The DAWN report. 1 in 10 energy drink-related emergency department visits results in hospitalization.

Chapter 46

Masley, S. (2005). *Ten years younger: The amazing ten week plan to look better, feel better, and turn back the clock.* New York: Broadway Books.

Palmer-Gierlinger, Mary Beth. CHC, AADP. Inspire Health Coaching, LLC.

Campbell, T.C. (2006). *The China study: Startling implications for diet, weight loss and long-term health.* Dallas: BenBella Books.

Chapter 47

Ward, B.W., Schiller, J.S., & Goodman, R.A. (2014). Multiple chronic conditions among US adults: A 2012 update. *Preventing Chronic Disease, 11,* 130389.

Chapter 49

Azarpazhooh, A., & Main, P.A. (2009). Efficacy of dental prophylaxis (rubber cup) for the prevention of caries and gingivitis: A systematic review of literature. *British Dental Journal, 207*(7), E14.

Redford-Badwal, D.A., & Hashim Nainar, S.M. (2002). Assessment of evidence-based dental prophylaxis education in postdoctoral pediatric dentistry programs. *Journal of Dental Education, 66*(9), 1044-8.

Steele, R.C., Waltner, L.A.W., & Bawden, J.W. (1984). The effect of tooth cleaning procedures on fluoride uptake in enamel. *American Academy of Pedodontics, 4,* Chapter 3.

Chapter 50

Pfaffe, T., Cooper-White, J., Beyerlein, P., et al. (2011). Diagnostic potential of saliva: Current state and future applications. *Clinical Chemistry, 57*(5), 675-87.

Mittal, S., Bansal, V., Garg., S., et al. (2011). The diagnostic role of saliva—A review. *Journal of Clinical and Experimental Dentistry, 3*(4), e314–e320.

National Institutes of Health. (2010, October). Fact sheet: Salivary diagnostics. Retrieved from http://report.nih.gov/nihfactsheets/ViewFactSheet.aspx?csid=65.

Wong, D. T. (2008). Salivary diagnostics. *American Scientist, 96*(1), 37.

Dentistry IQ. (2014, November 11). PeriRx's launch of SaliMark OSCC salivary test for oral cancer includes free CE course and more. Retrieved from http://www.dentistryiq.com/articles/2014/11/perirxs-launch-of-salimark-oscc-salivary-test-for-oral-cancer-includes-free-ce-course-and-more.html.

Chapter 52

American Heart Association. (2014). Heart disease and stroke statistics—2014 update: A report from the American Heart Association. *Circulation, 129*(3), 28-292.

Boyle, J.P., Thompson, T.J., Gregg, E.W., et al. (2010). Project of the year 2050 burden of diabetes in the U.S. adult population: Dynamic modeling of incidence, mortality and prediabetes prevalence. *Population Health Metrics, 8,* 29.

Heidenreich, P.A., Trogdon, J.G., Khavjou, O.A., et al. (2011). Forecasting the future of cardiovascular disease in the United States. *Circulation, 123*(8), 933-44.

U.S. National Research Council and U.S. Institute of Medicine. (2013). Woolf, S.H. and Aron, L. (Eds.) *U.S. health in international perspective: Shorter lives, poorer health.* Washington, D.C.: National Academies Press.

Chapter 55

Diamond, D. (2013, January 1). Just 8% of people achieve their New Year's resolutions. *Forbes* online. Retrieved from http://www.forbes.com/sites/dandiamond/2013/01/01/just-8-of-people-achieve-their-new-years-resolutions-heres-how-they-did-it/.

Remen, R.N. (1996). *Kitchen table wisdom: Stories that heal.* New York: Riverhead Books.

Blabber M🔘uth!

INDEX

Ghrelin, 113
Gingivitis, 13–16
  cause of, 14, 16
  during pregnancy, 100
  prevalence of, 1
  as prosthetic joint infection cause, 106
  signs and symptoms of, 13, 14, 48
  tooth brushing-based prevention of, 48
  treatment for, 15–16, 57
Glantz, Stanton, 229, 230
Glick, Michael, 294
Glucose, 29, 94, 232
Gluten sensitivity, 247
Grinding, of teeth. *See* Bruxism
Gum disease. *See* Periodontal disease
Gums
  anatomy of, 5
  bleeding/reddish, 5, 14, 15, 16, 43–44
  healthy, 18
  inflammation of, 14
  as protection against infection, 55
  recession of, 6, 28, 43–44
    aggressive tooth brushing-related,
        34, 190
    root decay-related, 35

H

Halitosis. *See* Bad breath
Han, Yiping W., 56, 100
Hard palate, anatomy of, 5
Headaches
  caffeine withdrawal-related, 242
  migraine, 244
  temporomandibular joint disorders-
        related, 176, 177–178
  tension-related, 7
Head and neck cancer, 126
Health
  effect of oral health on, 3–4
  individuals' responsibility for, 280–281
  key strategies for, 286–288
  national decline in, 277–281
Healthcare
  facilitated wellness model of, 284
  national expenditures for, 279

Healthcare crisis
  addictions-related, 213–214
  government's response to, 276, 293
  individuals' response to, 293–295
Healthcare team, criteria for selection of,
        251, 253–256, 257, 288
Health change behavior
  of friends and family, 289–292
  of individuals, 280–281
  within nation and communities, 293–295
  peer-based, 294
Heart attacks
  risk factors for
    coronary artery disease, 62
    oral bacteria, 56
    poor oral health, 47, 59–60, 61
Heartburn, 119, 120
Heart disease, 61-66
  genetic predisposition for, test for, 268,
        269
  as mortality cause, 59
  risk factors for, 59–60
    chronic systemic inflammation, 50
    diabetes, 79
    junk food, 246
    obesity, 92
    periodontitis, 67
    poor oral health, 47
    smoking, 224
Herpes simplex virus infection, 169–170
High-fructose corn syrup (HFCS), 232,
        235–236
High-sensitivity C-reactive protein test. *See*
        C-reactive protein test
HIV (human immunodeficiency virus)
        infection, 14, 126
Honey, 79–80
Hopkins, Claude, 195
Hormones, 95. *See also specific* hormones
  in pregnancy, 102
Hospital patients, respiratory disease
        prevention in, 87, 88, 89
Human Mouth as a Focus of Infection
        (Miller), 54

10 *Years Younger* (Masley), 247
Thich Nhat Hanh, 135
Throat
    anatomy of, 7
    size of opening in, 115
Throat cancer, 119, 120, 156, 225
Thrush, oral, 225
Tobacco. *See also* Smokeless tobacco;
        Smoking
    as dry mouth cause, 126, 128
Tongue
    anatomy of, 5
    brushing of, 165
    "hairy," 225
Tongue cancer, 70, 119, 120, 155, 156, 225
Tonsillar cancer, 156
Tonsils, anatomy of, 7
Toothache
    dying pulp-related, 38, 39
    root decay-related, 35
Tooth alteration, 147–151
Toothbrushes, 189–194
Tooth decay, 27-33. *See also* Root decay
    in children, 11, 27, 28
    as chronic disease cause, 27
    government program against, 229
    as heart attack risk factor, 63–64, 65
    in older adults, 27, 34
    prevention of, 41
        in children, 11
        with mouth rinses/washes, 205–206
    as respiratory disease risk factor, 87–88
    risk assessment for, 30–31
    risk factors for
        acid reflux, 120
        alcohol, 219
        depression, 140
        obesity, 96
        oral bacteria, 9, 56
        smoking, 225
        sugar, 233, 286
    warning signs of, 30
Tooth function, 17
Tooth lightening, 138, 143–146, 148
    with mouth rinses/washes, 206, 207

Tooth loss, 42–46
    complete (edentulism), 68
    effect on facial structure, 18
    as lung cancer risk factor, 70–71
    reimplantation of lost teeth, 44–45
    risk factors for, 43
        obesity, 96
        periodontal disease, 27
        periodontitis, 18, 19
        psychological disorders, 27
        root decay, 37
        tooth decay, 27
    warning signs of, 43–44
Toothpaste, 195-197
    allergens in, 14, 16
    cavity-preventing, 32, 33
    for dry mouth, 127, 128
    fluoride in, 211
    sodium lauryl sulfate in, 162–163
    whitening, 143–144
Twain, Mark, 226

U

Ulcers
 oral, 168–169, 171
 stomach, 67
Upper airway simulation (UAS) therapy,
        116–117
Uterus, oral bacteria-related infections of,
        102, 103
Uvula
    anatomy of, 5
    surgical removal of, 174

V

Veneers, 138, 150
Vermillion border, 4
    fading of, 162
Viruses. *See also* Human immunodeficiency
        virus (HIV) infection; Human
        papillomavirus (HPV) infection
    cancer-causing, 68
Vitamin D, 248–249